Student Laboratory Manual for

Seidel's Guide to

Physical Examination

Student Laboratory Manual for

Seidel's Guide to

Physical Examination

Eighth Edition

Jane W. Ball, DrPH, RN, CPNP
Trauma Systems Consultant
American College of Surgeons
Gaithersburg, Maryland

Joyce E. Dains, DrPH, JD, RN, FNP-BC
Advanced Practice Nursing Program Director
The University of Texas
M. D. Anderson Cancer Center
Houston, Texas

John A. Flynn, MD, MBA, MEd
Clinical Director and Professor of Medicine
Division of General Internal Medicine
The Johns Hopkins University
School of Medicine
Baltimore, Maryland

Barry S. Solomon, MD, MPH
Assistant Professor of Pediatrics
Medical Director, Harriet Lane Clinic
Division of General Pediatrics and Adolescent
Medicine
The Johns Hopkins University
School of Medicine
Baltimore, Maryland

Rosalyn W. Stewart, MD, MS, MBA
Assistant Professor of Pediatrics and Medicine
Department of Internal Pediatrics and Medicine
The Johns Hopkins University
School of Medicine
Baltimore, Maryland

Prepared By
Denise Vanacore-Chase, PHD, CRNP, ANP-BC
Director of Primary Health Care Services
Director, Nurse Practitioner Program and DNP
Program
Frances M. Maguire School of Nursing and
Health Professions
Gwynedd-Mercy University
Gwynedd Valley, Pennsylvania

Reviewed By
Alicia C. Henning, RN, BSM, SANE
Member of ACFEI: American College of Forensic
Examiners
Member of IAFN: International Association of
Forensic Nurses
Breckenridge Memorial Hospital
Hardinsburg, Kentucky

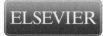

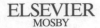

3251 Riverport Lane
St. Louis, Missouri 63043

STUDENT LABORATORY MANUAL FOR
SEIDEL'S GUIDE TO PHYSICAL EXAMINATION

ISBN: 978-0-323-16952-3

Executive Content Strategist: Kristin Geen
Content Manager: Jamie Randall
Associate Content Development Specialist: Melissa Rawe
Publishing Services Manager: Hemamalini Rajendrababu
Project Manager: Manchu Rajeev
Cover Designer: Gopalakrishnan Venkatram

Printed in the United States of America

Last digit is the print number: 9 8 7 6 5 4 3 2 1

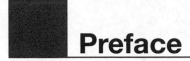

Preface

This *Student Laboratory Manual for Mosby's Guide to Physical Examination,* eighth edition, has been designed to help you achieve the goals associated with learning to interview patients for a health history and to perform physical examinations. Each chapter in the *Laboratory Manual* corresponds to one in the textbook, with the same title and chapter number. The correct answers to the questions are listed in the back of the *Laboratory Manual* and on the website so you can evaluate your comprehension of the material.

Each chapter in the *Laboratory Manual* begins with a list of Learning Objectives for use in assessing your comprehension of the material. A variety of exercises in each chapter helps you practice and confirm your understanding of the concepts, key terms, and techniques of examination. These exercises include the following:

- **Key Terms:** A list of key terms from the textbook chapter with the accompanying definitions to apply to the other exercises in the manual.
- **Concepts Application:** Exercises will help you evaluate and assess examination findings to interpret the results and recognize normal and abnormal outcomes.
- **Case Study:** Case Studies give you the opportunity to apply data evaluation skills in a clinical setting. Additional information or data needed to further determine a diagnosis or course of action may be called for, and you will have the opportunity to suggest further examination.
- **Critical Thinking:** Problems are posed to give you practice in analyzing patient information and managing interactions with patients
- **Content Review Questions:** Multiple-choice, fill-in-the-blank, and matching questions will help you review the primary concepts and terminology related to the content. Anatomic drawings to be labeled will challenge you to apply knowledge associated with the relevant body systems.

It is my hope that the *Laboratory Manual* will be helpful to you in your study of physical examination.

Denise Vanacore-Chase,
PhD, CRNP, ANP-BC

Contents

1 The History and Interviewing Process

LEARNING OBJECTIVES

After studying Chapter 1 in the textbook and completing this section of the laboratory manual, students should be able to:

1. Recognize ethical considerations in patient–examiner relationships.
2. Classify aspects of communication that affect the interview process.
3. Obtain a comprehensive health history.
4. Apply the elements of a clinical presentation to a health history.
5. Organize data according to a clinical history outline.
6. Differentiate between the history and interviewing process used for an adult patient with the process used for patients of special populations such as patients with disabilities, pregnant patients, and frail patients.

TEXTBOOK REVIEW

Chapter 1: The History and Interviewing Process (pp. 1–20)

CHAPTER OVERVIEW

This chapter explores the development of your relationships with patients and the building of the histories of your patients. Because you and each patient are involved in a joint effort, the formation of the health history as "building" a history rather than "taking" one reflects each patient's perspectives and unique status. Effective techniques for developing a patient relationship and facilitating communication with each patient are reviewed. An in-depth discussion of the components and structure of the health history is included. The history is vital to the interpretation of the physical examination. Finally, this chapter offers widely accepted, time-tested approaches to the structure of a history with adaptations suggested for patients of both genders and with disabilities.

TERMINOLOGY REVIEW

CAGE—questionnaire for discussing the use of alcohol, which includes cutting down (C), annoyance by criticism (A), guilty (G), and eye openers (E).

Chief concern (CC)—a brief statement of the reason the patient is seeking care.

Family history (FH)—blood relatives in the immediate or extended family with illnesses that have features similar to the patient's concern.

Functional assessment—questions concerning the ability to take care of one's daily needs that are part of the review of systems.

History of present illness (HPI)—a step-by-step evaluation of the circumstances that surround the primary reason for the patient's visit.

Intimate partner violence (IPV)—includes a range of abusive behaviors perpetrated by someone who is or was involved in an intimate relationship with the victim.

Past medical history (PMH)—the patient's state of overall health before the present problem.

Personal and social history (SH)—work, marriage, sexual, and spiritual experiences; the patient's use of alcohol, tobacco, and drugs.

Review of systems (ROS)—identifies the presence or absence of health-related issues in each body system.

Symptom analysis—questions specifying the onset, location, duration, intensity, characteristics, and aggravating and alleviating factors.

Clinical Case Study

Rachael Roman is a 25-year-old woman who presents to your office with a complaint of fatigue. She is a college graduate, but she is currently working as a waitress because she has not been able to secure a job in her field.

1. What is this patient's chief complaint?

2. What questions would you ask to complete the HPI?

3. What systems should you ask questions about during the ROS?

Concepts Application

Listed below are patient behaviors that can create tension for the examiner. For each patient behavior listed, provide a behavior by the examiner that could help decrease the tension. (Write your answers in the space provided in the right column.)

Patient Behavior	Examiner Behavior to Decrease Tension
Seduction	
Depression	
Anxiety	
Excessive flattery	
Financial concerns	
Silence	

Critical Thinking Case Study 1

Reed Smith is a 35-year-old man who presents to your office with a complaint of left foot pain. He describes this as a severe burning pain on the outside edge of the heel of his left foot. The pain is worse in the morning and when he walks barefoot. The pain improves when he applies ice to his foot. In addition, the patient states, "I have been using Tylenol one or two times per day." The pain started 2 weeks ago after the patient was walking on the beach. The pain lasts for 2 to 3 hours in the morning and then seems to subside after he is up and walking for a while.

1. Based on the information in this case study, identify each of the following characteristics of the patient's pain using the mnemonic device "OLDCARTS."

   Onset:

   Location:

   Duration:

   Characteristics:

   Aggravating factors:

   Relieving factors:

   Timing:

   Severity:

Critical Thinking Case Study 2

Marci Jones is a 52-year-old woman who presents to your office with sudden burning and stabbing pain in the left orbit. She says her pain is severe, and she is outwardly agitated. She experienced similar pain the day before at about the same time. She denies associated signs or symptoms of nausea or vomiting, aura, new medications, and excessive alcohol use. She reports a 24-year pack history for smoking and says she has high stress on her job, does daily exercise, and follows a prudent diet. PMH is unremarkable with the exception of "spells" of headaches similar to this from time to time. According to the patient, these symptoms occur without warning and resolve after a few hours but usually return the next day. This may go on for a week or more before the symptoms stop until the next episode begins.

1. What components of a health history are present in this case study?

2. What components should have been added to the health history?

3. What components are only partially complete?

CONTENT REVIEW QUESTIONS

Multiple Choice

Circle the correct answer for each of the following questions.

1. Which of the following will best facilitate the interview when obtaining a history for a deaf patient who can read lips?
   a. Speaking loudly
   b. Using gestures
   c. Speaking slowly
   d. Sitting to the side of the patient

2. Approximately what percentage of patients interviewed have a sexual orientation other than heterosexual?
   a. 2%
   b. 5%
   c. 10%
   d. 20%

3. During a history, the patient indicates he has an uncle and a brother with sickle cell disease. Which of the following is an appropriate method to document this information?
   a. Document this as chief complaint.
   b. Include it in the family history.
   c. Include this in past medical history.
   d. Incorporate this information in the social history.

4. Which approach is recommended at the onset of an interview?
   a. Use a structured approach to ask questions.
   b. Introduce yourself and include a detailed description of your background and qualifications.
   c. Use an open-ended approach; let the patient explain the problem or reason for the visit.
   d. Start with the family history and past medical history to determine the underlying problem.

5. Which of the following questions may lead to an inaccurate patient response?
   a. "Where do you feel the pain?"
   b. "How does this situation make you feel?"
   c. "What happened after you noticed your injury?"
   d. "That was a horrible experience, wasn't it?"

6. Repeating a patient's answer is an attempt to
   a. confirm an accurate understanding.
   b. discourage patient anger or hostility.
   c. teach the patient new medical terms.
   d. test the patient's knowledge.

7. Which of the following history types is unique to a pediatric history?
   a. Family history
   b. Developmental history
   c. Social history
   d. Past medical history

8. When interviewing an adolescent who is reluctant to talk during an interview, it is best to
   a. tell the patient you must have honest answers to your questions.
   b. ensure confidentiality regarding information discussed.
   c. inform the patient that adolescents often have trouble expressing their feelings.
   d. obtain the history from a parent or other family member.

9. During an interview, your patient admits to feeling worthless and having a sleep disturbance for the past 3 weeks. These are clues that warrant the exploration of
   a. risk for suicide.
   b. split personality.
   c. cognitive function.
   d. functional assessment.

10. Mrs. Carol Turner is a 38-year-old mother who brings her 1-year-old son in for health care. Which of the following requests to the child's mother would be most appropriate for the interviewer to make at the beginning of the interview?
    a. "Mom, please place your son in your lap."
    b. "Carol, please place your son in your lap."
    c. "Mrs. Turner, please place your son in your lap."
    d. "Sweetie, please place your son in your lap."

11. Which type of questionnaire concerning drug and alcohol use is advocated, although not clinically validated, for adolescent patients?
    a. TACE
    b. CAGE
    c. CRAFFT
    d. DDST

12. Jerry, a 26-year-old homosexual man, is having a health history taken. Which question regarding sexual activity would most likely *hamper* trust between Jerry and the interviewer?
    a. "Are you married, or do you have a girlfriend?"
    b. "Tell me about your living situation."
    c. "Are you sexually active?"
    d. "Are your partners men, women, or both?"

13. A conversation with a parent concerning a 5-year-old child
    a. violates the child's need for privacy.
    b. is inappropriate because the child is able to talk with you.
    c. provides significant information about family dynamics.
    d. causes distrust in the child toward the examiner.

14. Long periods of silence during an interview may indicate
    a. a need for the health care provider to increase the pace of the interview.
    b. an inability of the patient to communicate.
    c. time needed to gain courage to discuss a painful topic.
    d. a need to terminate the interview because of the patient's inability to pay attention.

15. When questioning a patient regarding a sensitive issue, such as drug use, it is best to
    a. begin by describing to the patient the effects of drug abuse on health.
    b. be direct, firm, and to the point.
    c. explain that the information will be shared only with health care workers.
    d. apologize to the patient for asking personal questions.

16. Direct questions are designed to
    a. attack sensitive material head on.
    b. demonstrate to the patient who is in charge of the interview process.
    c. ensure confidentiality.
    d. obtain or clarify specific details about an answer.

17. Interviewers should identify and assess their own feelings, such as hostility and prejudice, in order to
    a. avoid inappropriate behavior.
    b. explain their biases to patients.
    c. express their idiosyncrasies.
    d. reduce communication barriers.

18. During an interview, a patient describes abdominal pain that often awakens him at night. Which of the following responses by the interviewer would facilitate the interviewing process?
    a. "Constipation can cause abdominal pain."
    b. "Do you need a sleeping medication?"
    c. "Pain is always worse at night, isn't it?"
    d. "Tell me what you mean by *often*."

19. When taking a patient's history, you are asked questions about your personal life. What is the best response to facilitate the interviewing process?
   a. Answer briefly and then refocus to the patient's history.
   b. Give as much detail as possible about the asked information.
   c. Ignore the question and continue with the patient's history.
   d. Tell the patient that it is inappropriate to answer personal questions.

20. During an interview, the patient describes problems associated with an illness and begins to cry. The best action in this situation is to
   a. stop the interview and reschedule for another time.
   b. allow the patient to cry and then resume when the patient is ready.
   c. change the topic to something less upsetting.
   d. continue the interview while the patient cries in order to get through it quickly.

2 Cultural Competency

LEARNING OBJECTIVES

After studying Chapter 2 in the textbook and completing this section of the laboratory manual, students should be able to:
1. Define cultural competence, cultural humility, and cultural awareness.
2. Examine differences and similarities between ethnic and physical characteristics.
3. Analyze the impact of culture on illness, health beliefs, and practices.
4. Examine modes of communication that explore a patient's culture.
5. Compare and contrast value orientations among cultural groups.

TEXTBOOK REVIEW

Chapter 2: Cultural Competency (pp. 21–29)

CHAPTER OVERVIEW

This chapter examines the definitions of cultural competence, cultural awareness, and cultural humility. In addition, the impact of cultural response and the components that affect the clinician's health assessment are reviewed. These components include modes of communication, health beliefs and practices, diet and nutritional practices, and the nature of relationships within the family. Finally, this chapter examines culturally competent health care providers and the need to adapt to the unique needs of patients of all backgrounds and cultures.

TERMINOLOGY REVIEW

Culture—reflects the whole human behavior, including ideas, and attitudes.
Cultural awareness—the deliberate self-examination of one's biases, stereotypes, prejudices, and assumptions about cultures that are different from one's own.
Cultural desire—motivation of a health care professional to "want to" engage in the process of becoming culturally competent.
Cultural humility—the ability to recognize one's limitations in knowledge and cultural perspective.
Cultural impact—the provision of health care services that is impacted by racial and ethnic differences.
Cultural knowledge—the process of seeking and obtaining a sound educational base about culturally and ethnically diverse groups.
Culturally competent care—sensitivity to the patient's heritage, sexual orientation, socioeconomic situation, ethnicity, and cultural background.
Cultural skill—the ability to collect culturally relevant data regarding the patient's presenting problem.
Race—a physical characteristic not based on culture.
Stereotype—an inflexible generalization about a group.

Clinical Case Study

Mrs. Howdruy is a 52-year-old Chinese woman who presents to your practice with a complaint of burning pain in the abdomen that occurs three to four times per week. She speaks very little English and arrives without her family to assist with communication.

1. What questions could you ask that explore the patient's culture?

2. What question could you ask the patient to find out about any treatment(s) she has already tried?

3. If Mrs. Howdruy practices the hot and cold belief system, what might she have tried as a self-treatment for her abdominal pain?

Concepts Application

Relate each of the following value orientations to a clinical scenario.

1. **Present oriented.** A patient is given the diagnosis of hypercholesterolemia. He is told by his clinician to watch his diet to lower his blood cholesterol. Assuming the patient is present oriented, what might be his response?

2. **Future oriented.** An overweight patient has diabetes mellitus. She is advised to lose 50 lb and to decrease the carbohydrates and increase the vegetables in her diet to lower her blood sugar. Assuming the patient is future oriented, what might be her response?

CRITICAL THINKING

Critical Thinking Case Study 1

Mr. Santiago is a 45-year-old Hispanic man who presents to your office with a complaint of sore throat, fever, and fatigue. You make the diagnosis of infectious mononucleosis and recommend that he take 2 weeks off from work.

1. What value orientation might this patient have that would affect his feelings about staying home from work because of his illness?

2. Because Mr. Santiago is Hispanic, his belief system may include the need for a balance between hot and cold. What hot and cold remedies might he have tried already to self-treat his condition?

Critical Thinking Case Study 2

You are caring for a minority patient who has a chronic illness requiring dietary teaching and education about medications. Listed below are areas for cultural assessment. For each area, list at least one question you could ask as part of a cultural assessment to better prepare for this patient's care.

1. Health beliefs and practices

2. Religious and ritual influences

3. Dietary practices

4. Family relationships and relational orientation

Self Reflection

Reflect on your care of patients of different cultures. What were your strengths in providing culturally competent care? What barriers to providing culturally competent care did you encounter? How did you manage your differences?

CONTENT REVIEW QUESTIONS

Multiple Choice

Circle the correct answer for each of the following questions.

1. Developing cultural sensitivity is vital in order for the examiner to be successful in
   a. performing a physical examination.
   b. recognizing and accepting health beliefs that differ from his or her own beliefs.
   c. identifying patients at high risk for various diseases.
   d. applying statistical trends of various ethnic and cultural groups.

2. The balance of hot and cold and its relationship to wellness is a concept that
   a. has been proven to be without validity.
   b. is common only in underdeveloped nations.
   c. has led to poor sanitization practice in many areas of the world.
   d. is believed by members of many cultures, including Arabs, Asians, Filipinos, and Hispanics.

3. Developing a knowledge base about cultural groups allows the practitioner to
   a. predict with complete accuracy the behavior and attitude of the patient.
   b. use stereotypic judgments to anticipate the patient's need for instruction and support.
   c. understand the behaviors, practices, and problems observed.
   d. change the behavior or practices of the patient to conform to health care practice.

4. Which of the following is an example of a cultural characteristic?
   a. Skin color
   b. Intelligence
   c. Skull size
   d. Shared belief

5. An integral part of the overall effort to respond adequately to a person in need is
   a. cultural awareness.
   b. ethnocentric bias.
   c. political correctness.
   d. racial alertness.

6. A young mother brings her infant to the emergency department with a high temperature and dehydration. Which of the following questions asked by an examiner demonstrates cultural awareness?
   a. "When did the symptoms begin?"
   b. "What do you think is causing this illness?"
   c. "Has your child been exposed to any sick children recently?"
   d. "What have you already done at home to manage your child's illness?"

7. Which group is most likely to be subjected to invasive cardiac procedures in the United States?
   a. Middle-class black individuals
   b. White men
   c. Upper class women
   d. Lower class Asians

8. A common mistake made by health care professionals is to
   a. acknowledge the practice of folk or herbal remedies.
   b. adapt health care concepts to meet the needs of individuals of other cultures.
   c. stereotype individuals based on color or ethnic group.
   d. carefully assess the understanding and beliefs of culturally diverse individuals.

9. All of the following are cultural considerations that affect health care *except*
   a. eye color, temperature, and visual acuity.
   b. social class, age, and gender.
   c. ethnic traditions, level of education, and family relationships.
   d. religious beliefs, dietary habits, and mode of communication.

10. Which of the following is an example of a physical, as opposed to a cultural, characteristic?
    a. Language
    b. Hair style
    c. Skin color
    d. Religious affiliation

11. Despite repeated instruction over a period of 3 years, the mother of three young children has still not had her children immunized. Which of the following questions would help the health care provider understand this situation?
    a. "When are you going to get your children immunized?"
    b. "What are your beliefs about immunizations?"
    c. "We have asked you to get your children immunized. Why has this not been done?"
    d. "Don't you understand that your children may get ill without immunizations?"

12. Which of the following beliefs is characteristic of a present-oriented individual?
    a. The individual understands the connection between past events and behaviors and future outcomes.
    b. The individual anticipates a brighter future and values change as a coping style.
    c. The individual maintains behaviors that were meaningful in the past (e.g., worshiping ancestors).
    d. The individual accepts each day as it comes and sees the future as unpredictable.

13. Which mode of communication may be offensive to a patient whose cultural perspective differs from that of the practitioner?
    a. Speaking in modulated tones
    b. Allowing quiet time for reflection during an interview
    c. Using reflection to repeat and clarify the information
    d. Maintaining firm and direct eye contact

14. Which of the following statements is an accurate interpretation of the concept of balancing hot and cold?
    a. Treatment to restore hot and cold balance requires the use of opposites
    b. The recommended treatment for a "cold" condition is to serve cold foods
    c. The recommended treatment for a "hot" condition is hot foods and cold medications
    d. Ailments and treatments considered "hot" or "cold" are related to the effect of body temperature

Examination Techniques and Equipment

LEARNING OBJECTIVES

After studying Chapter 3 in the textbook and completing this section of the laboratory manual, students should be able to:

1. Apply standard precautions for infection control to the examination process.
2. Correctly obtain baseline data (vital signs, height, and weight) and describe the meaning of the findings.
3. Differentiate various types of equipment used for physical examination.
4. Describe the purpose of various types of equipment used for physical examination.
5. Demonstrate the correct use of various types of equipment used for physical examination.
6. Identify various techniques applied during a physical examination.
7. Describe the purpose of various techniques used during a physical examination.
8. Demonstrate correct application of the various techniques used during physical examination.

TEXTBOOK REVIEW

Chapter 3: Examination Techniques and Equipment (pp. 30–49)

CHAPTER OVERVIEW

This chapter provides an overview of the techniques of inspection, palpation, percussion, and auscultation that are used throughout the physical examination. The correct application for each technique is reviewed. Necessary precautions to prevent infection are identified. The chapter also reviews the various types of equipment used for physical examination and describes their correct use.

TERMINOLOGY REVIEW

Amsler grid—a device used to screen patients at risk for macular degeneration.
Aperture setting—a function that adjusts or changes light variations of an ophthalmoscope for examination; the large aperture is the one used most often.
Auscultation—listening for sounds produced by the body.
Axillary infrared thermometer—for neonates, suitable for use in incubators and under radiate warmers.
Bell of stethoscope—the part of the stethoscope that detects low-frequency sounds.
Calipers—designed to measure the thickness of subcutaneous tissue at certain points of the body.
Dermatoscope—a skin surface microscope used to inspect the surface of pigmented skin lesions.
Diaphragm of stethoscope—the part of the stethoscope that detects high-pitched sounds.
Doppler—technology that amplifies sounds by use of ultrasonic waves.
"E" chart—a tool used to test visual acuity, especially useful for patients who cannot read or speak English.
Goniometer—an instrument used to determine the degree of flexion or extension of a joint.
Graves speculum—a speculum with a bottom blade slightly longer than the top blade.
Inspection—the process of observation of the patient.
Monofilament—a single strand of fiber used to assess sensation to the plantar surface of the foot.
Nasal speculum—an instrument that is used with a pen light to visualize the lower and middle turbinates of the nose.
Near-vision chart (Rosenbaum)—used for screening near vision.
Neurologic hammer—an instrument with a brush and a sharp needle in the base and head.
Ophthalmoscope—an instrument that allows the examiner to evaluate the internal eye structures.
Otoscope—an instrument that allows the examiner to evaluate the internal ear structures.
Palpation—use of the hands and fingers to gather information through the sense of touch.
Panoptic ophthalmoscope—the panoramic ophthalmoscope head uses an optical design that allows a larger field of view.
Pederson speculum—a speculum used for women with small vaginal openings.
Percussion—involves striking one object against another to produce vibration and subsequent sound waves.
Percussion reflex hammer—instrument used to test deep tendon reflexes.

11

Pulse oximeter—instrument that measures the percentage of hemoglobin saturated with oxygen.
Scoliometer—instrument that measures the degree of rotation of the spine to screen for scoliosis.
Snellen chart—a tool used to test visual acuity for literate English-speaking patients.
Strabismoscope—an instrument that uses a one-way mirror to detect subtle eye movements.
Sphygmomanometer—an instrument that measures blood pressure; it can be electronic, aneroid, or mercury style.
Thermometer—instrument used for determining temperature; it can be oral, rectal, axillary, or tympanic.
Transilluminator—an instrument that differentiates tissue, fluid, and air within a body cavity.
Tuning fork—an instrument used for screening tests for auditory function and for vibratory sensation.
Tympanometer—an instrument used to assess function of the inner ear.
Wood's lamp—a black light used to detect fungal infections or corneal abrasion.

APPLICATION TO CLINICAL PRACTICE

Clinical Concepts Application 1

For each description listed below, provide the name of the examination technique or equipment described. (Write your answers in the space provided in the right column.)

Description	Examination Technique or Equipment
Gathering information through touch	
Grid used to assess for macular degeneration	
The fifth vital sign	
Source of light with a narrow beam	
Used to test deep tendon reflexes	
Used to visualize turbinates	
Assesses near vision	
Measures skinfold thickness	
Larger field of view in eye examination	

Clinical Concepts Application 2

Complete the following table by providing the expected examination findings. (Write your answers in the space provided in the right column.)

Area Percussed	Percussion Tone Expected
Stomach	
Sternum	
Lung of patient with emphysema	
Liver	
Lung of patient with pneumonia	
Lung of normal patient	
Abdomen with large tumor	

CRITICAL THINKING

1. Mrs. Johnson is 72 years old and is brought to the clinic by her daughter. She has an abdominal fistula that is draining foul, purulent fluid. She also has bowel and urinary incontinence. What infection control measures should be implemented for Mrs. Johnson?

2. Explain (a) when a non-antimicrobial soap can be used and (b) when an antimicrobial soap is indicated to wash one's hands.

3. Charles Helms comes to the diabetic clinic. He has not been to the clinic in a very long time and tells you he has some problems with his feet. "They just don't feel right," he says.

   a. What types of questions are appropriate to ask Mr. Helms regarding this symptom?

   b. Based on the patient's statement, "They just don't feel right," what are the areas of concern, and how can this be assessed during and examination?

CONTENT REVIEW QUESTIONS

Multiple Choice
Circle the correct answer for each of the following questions.

1. Which of the following infection control guidelines are currently recommended by the Centers for Disease Control and Prevention (CDC)?
   a. Universal precautions
   b. Body substance isolation
   c. Standard precautions
   d. Illness-based precautions

2. A patient presents with multiple raised lesions on her skin. Which instrument should be used to examine these lesions?
   a. Calipers
   b. Ruler
   c. Tympanometer
   d. Transilluminator

3. In an outpatient setting such as a clinic, how should infection control practice differ from that in the acute-care setting?
   a. The use of transmission-based precautions is not applicable in an outpatient setting.
   b. Infection control is limited to protecting outpatient health care providers.
   c. The spread of infection to other patients is not a concern in the outpatient setting.
   d. Infection control practice is applicable in all health care settings.

4. In which of the following situations is transillumination an appropriate examination technique?
   a. Assessment of vesicles on the skin
   b. Detection of fluid within the sinuses
   c. Measurement of bone density in the skull
   d. Determination of a mass in the abdomen

5. Which of the following instruments is used in conjunction with a simple nasal speculum to visualize the lower and middle turbines of the nose?
    a. Otoscope
    b. Penlight
    c. Ophthalmoscope
    d. Goniometer

6. On first meeting, the examiner notices that the patient has an obvious odor. Which examination technique is the examiner using in this scenario?
    a. Inspection
    b. Palpation
    c. Percussion
    d. Auscultation

7. Focused visual attention obtains data from
    a. inspection.
    b. palpation.
    c. percussion.
    d. auscultation.

8. Which technique is applied throughout the entire examination and interview process?
    a. Inspection
    b. Palpation
    c. Percussion
    d. Auscultation

9. As a component of palpation, which surface is most sensitive to vibration?
    a. Fingertips
    b. Heel of the hand
    c. Dorsal surface of the hand
    d. Ulnar surface of the hand

10. How deep should the examiner's hands press while performing deep palpation?
    a. 1 cm
    b. 2 cm
    c. 4 cm
    d. 8 cm

11. The term *intensity*, when used in relation to percussion tones, refers to
    a. the loudness of the tone.
    b. the location of the tone.
    c. the musical quality of the tone.
    d. the length of duration the tone is heard.

12. Indirect finger percussion involves striking the middle finger of the nondominant hand with:
    a. the fist.
    b. a percussion hammer.
    c. the tip of the middle finger of the dominant hand.
    d. a stethoscope.

13. A patient has a urinary tract infection. The examiner wishes to assess tenderness over the kidney. Which examination technique is appropriate?
    a. Light finger palpation over the kidney
    b. Firm fist percussion over the kidney
    c. Deep abdominal palpation of the kidney
    d. Auscultation for kidney bruit

14. The examiner has detected a superficial mass in the skin. What part of the hand is best to use to palpate this mass?
    a. Fingertips
    b. Heel of the hand
    c. Dorsal surface of the hand
    d. Ulnar surface of the hand

15. Ideally, auscultation should be carried out last, *except* when examining the
    a. lungs.
    b. heart.
    c. abdomen.
    d. kidney.

16. Which of the following techniques is *incorrect* and affects the accuracy of auscultation?
    a. Placing the stethoscope firmly on the surface to be auscultated
    b. Auscultating through clothing
    c. Isolating one sound at a time during auscultation
    d. Listening for sound characteristics

17. When measuring the length of an infant, the measurement should extend from the
    a. forehead to feet.
    b. crown to tip of toes in a prone position.
    c. head to toes in an upright position.
    d. crown to heel in a supine position.

18. The tubing of a stethoscope should be less than 18 inches long to prevent
    a. transmission of external noise.
    b. tangling of the tubing in the examiner's clothing or pockets.
    c. distortion of sounds during auscultation.
    d. magnification of the transmitted sounds.

19. Which of the following is true regarding the correct use of a stethoscope?
    a. The bell is pressed lightly against the skin to detect low-frequency sounds.
    b. The bell is pressed firmly against the skin to hear low-frequency sounds.
    c. The diaphragm is pressed firmly against the skin to hear low-frequency sounds.
    d. The diaphragm is pressed lightly against the skin to hear high-frequency sounds.

20. The examiner must be sure that the earpieces of the stethoscope are placed so that the alignment fits the contour of the ear canal. In which direction should they be placed?
    a. Pointing upward
    b. Pointing downward
    c. Pointing forward
    d. Pointing backward

21. In which of the following situations is use of a Doppler indicated?
    a. Measurement of body temperature in a hypothermic patient
    b. Auscultation of the abdomen in a patient with hypoactive or absent bowel sounds
    c. Measurement of blood pressure in a patient with hypertension
    d. Auscultation of a nonpalpable pulse in a patient with peripheral vascular disease

22. The red numbers on a lens selector dial of an ophthalmoscope indicate
    a. that a large amount of light will enter the eye being examined.
    b. that a small amount of light will enter the eye being examined.
    c. positive magnification.
    d. negative magnification.

23. While performing an internal eye examination, the examiner observes a fundal lesion. What feature on the ophthalmoscope permits the examiner to estimate the size and location of the lesion?
    a. Grid light
    b. Slit light
    c. Red-free light
    d. Small light

24. An ophthalmoscope has positive and negative magnification in order to
    a. compensate for myopia or hyperopia in the examiner's or the patient's eyes.
    b. allow for magnification of both the anterior eye and the posterior eye.
    c. compensate for the degree of dilation of the patient's eyes.
    d. allow for visualization of the eye in patients with normal vision and in those with glaucoma.

25. In which of the following situations is the pneumatic attachment of an otoscope indicated?
    a. Removal of excessive ear wax from an adult or child
    b. Inflation of the ear canal for improved viewing in an adult with a collapsed canal
    c. Assessment of pressure behind the tympanic membrane of a child
    d. Evaluation of the cone of light reflex in an adult or child

26. The difference between a tuning fork for auditory screening and one for vibratory sensation is
    a. the sound frequency generated.
    b. the strike force applied by the examiner on the forks.
    c. the length of the tuning forks.
    d. the auditory screening fork is electric, but the vibratory fork is not.

27. Very young children may feel threatened by the use of a reflex hammer during examination. What could the examiner use in place of a reflex hammer that would be less threatening?
    a. Tuning fork
    b. Tongue blade
    c. End of a stethoscope
    d. Examiner's finger

28. According to the Centers for Disease Control and Prevention, the health care provider should apply infection control measures when caring for which group of patients?
    a. Patients with known infectious diseases
    b. Patients with possible infectious diseases
    c. Patients who appear ill
    d. All patients regardless of their infectious status

Vital Signs and Pain Assessment

LEARNING OBJECTIVES

After studying Chapter 4 in the textbook and completing this section of the laboratory manual, students should be able to:

1. Examine the assessment of vital signs and pain in adult patients as well as in special populations such as infants, children, and older adults.
2. Describe the techniques to assess vital signs including temperature, pulse, respirations, and blood pressure.
3. Discuss the use of pain assessment scales in the history and physical examination of pain.
4. Evaluate vital sign findings that deviate from normal.
5. Analyze the impact of pain on physiologic responses.
6. Describe a focused history and physical examination in a patient experiencing an alteration in vital signs or pain.

TEXTBOOK REVIEW

Chapter 4: Vital Signs and Pain Assessment (pp. 50–63)

CHAPTER OVERVIEW

This chapter focuses on the assessment of vital signs and pain in adult patients and in special populations, including infants, children, and older adults. Use of the health history to elicit data about the patient's vital signs and pain is reviewed, and specific evaluation of the pain is discussed. This chapter also reviews pain patterns and pain assessment skills that may be used to assess the patient's pain. Finally, this chapter applies the physical examination to specific findings related to pain.

TERMINOLOGY REVIEW

Blood pressure (BP)—the force of the blood against the wall of an artery as the ventricles of the heart contract and relax.
Complex regional pain syndrome—the presence of regional pain beyond the original nerve injury with motor, sensory, and autonomic changes after a predominately traumatic, noxious event, with or without specific nerve injury.
Checklist of nonverbal pain indicators—a pain scale for older adults.
Korotkoff sounds—turbulence of blood flow in the artery.
Neonatal infant pain scale—a pain scale for infants.
Neuropathic pain—a form of chronic pain cause by a primary lesion or by dysfunction of the central nervous system that persists longer than expected after healing.
Numeric pain intensity scale—a pain scale for verbal older children, adolescents, and adults.
Oucher scale—a pain scale for children.
Premature infant pain profile—a pain scale for premature infants.
Pulse rate—palpated over an artery close to the body surface that lies over bones.
Pulse pressure—the difference between the systolic and diastolic pressures.
Pyrexia—the fever response is triggered by the production of prostaglandins.
Respiratory rate—assesses the respiratory rate by inspecting the rise and fall of the chest; the expected adult rate is 12 to 20 breaths/min.
Temperature—temperature assessment is most commonly performed by oral, rectal, axillary, or tympanic routes.
The Painometer—a multidimensional measure of pain.
Wong/Baker faces rating scale—a pain scale for children.

Clinical Case Study 1

Mrs. King is a 41-year-old woman who presents to the clinic with complaints of a temperature. She does not have any past medical illnesses. She does not smoke or drink alcohol.

1. What questions would you ask Mrs. King to evaluate her present fever problem?

2. What questions regarding associated symptoms would you ask Mrs. King?

3. What medications questions would you ask Mrs. King?

Clinical Case Study 2

Mrs. Brooks is a 65-year-old woman who is hospitalized for her cardiac dysrhythmia. Her history includes carpal tunnel syndrome, gastroesophageal reflux disease (GERD), and osteoarthritis.

1. What pain findings would you expect for each diagnosis listed below? (Write your answers in the space provided in the right column.)

Diagnosis	Pain Findings
General pain	
Carpal tunnel	
GERD	
Osteoarthritis	

CRITICAL THINKING

Critical Thinking Case Study 1

Mr. Kasher is a 65-year-old man who is brought to the office for hypertension follow-up. On presentation, his BP is 148/92 mm Hg and pulse is 56 beats/min.

1. What is the most common cause of hypertension in elderly adults?

2. What is the rationale for the change in pulse?

Critical Thinking Case Study 2

Mrs. Timony is an 85-year-old patient who presents to your clinic with a complaint of "soreness" in the abdomen.

1. What physical signs would you expect to find during a physical examination of Mrs. Timony?

2. If Mrs. Timony complains of cramping sensations. What would you anticipate her underlying condition to be?

CONTENT REVIEW QUESTIONS

Multiple Choice

Circle the correct answer for each of the following questions.

1. Mrs. Kaymos is a 32-year-old postoperative patient who has undergone an appendectomy. When assessing your patient, you should remember
   a. the patient's previous experiences with pain.
   b. that the intensity of pain is easily determined.
   c. that dementia is a response to excessive pain.
   d. that pain is an objective symptom.

2. Mr. Greenspan is an 87-year-old man who is hospitalized with complaints of abdominal pain. Which of the following is true?
   a. Assessment of aggravating factors is the most critical assessment finding.
   b. Older patients should be asked about pain in the past tense.
   c. Delirium occurs in 85% of hospitalized patients.
   d. Dementia occurs in 50% of older adults in hospitals.

3. Which term would be most commonly used by a child expressing pain?
   a. Aching
   b. Hurt
   c. Sore
   d. Stabbing

4. Mrs. Snyder is a 32-year-old patient who is admitted for a right fractured ankle after an automobile accident. Which of the following would you not expect to find on assessment of Mrs. Snyder's pain?
   a. Facial distortions such as grimacing
   b. Changes in vital signs, including BP and pulse
   c. Increase in attention span and talking
   d. Splinting of her leg and ankle

5. Children experience pain just as much as adults do. At about what age is a child able respond to a pediatric pain scale?
   a. 3 years old
   b. 7 years old
   c. 11 years old
   d. 14 years old

6. When you are giving an injection to an infant, which of the following would decrease the pain?
   a. Holding the infant gently
   b. After the injection, putting ice on the site
   c. Giving the infant a pacifier
   d. Administering sugar water

7. When you are completing an assessment on a patient with pain, it is important to
   a. do a complete assessment to check for referred pain.
   b. learn the patient's customary terminology.
   c. medicate the patient before the assessment so as not to hurt the patient.
   d. always use a nonverbal patient pain scale.

8. The "gold standard" in pain assessment is the patient's
   a. nonverbal communication.
   b. perception of his or her own pain.
   c. vital signs.
   d. fear of addiction.

9. Mr. Respin is a 51-year-old patient admitted with burning, shocklike pain in his left hand. This finding would indicate
   a. nerve tissue damage.
   b. cardiac pain.
   c. bone and soft tissue pain.
   d. visceral pain.

10. How does an examiner determine the correct size of a BP cuff on an adult? The cuff should
    a. be 2½ to 3 times the length of the arm.
    b. be able to wrap around the arm once.
    c. cover 25% of the upper arm.
    d. be 40% of the circumference of the arm.

11. How is a BP reading affected if an adult cuff is used on a small child?
    a. BP readings will be falsely low.
    b. BP readings will be falsely high.
    c. Results will demonstrate a false high systolic reading and a false low diastolic reading
    d. BP readings are not affected; cuff size is merely a matter of comfort.

12. Axillary measurement of temperature correlates best with core temperatures of
    a. infants.
    b. toddlers.
    c. adolescents.
    d. adults.

13. The usual respiratory rate for children age 6 years old is
    a. 20 to 40 breaths/min.
    b. 20 to 30 breaths/min.
    c. 16 to 22 breaths/min.
    d. 12 to 20 breaths/min.

14. You are caring for a 10-year-old boy. What would the normal heart rate be for this child?
    a. 80 to 120 beats/min
    b. 75 to 115 beats/min
    c. 70 to 110 beats/min
    d. 60 to 110 beats/min

15. Ricky is a 14-year-old adolescent who presents to the office with his mother. His mom states that he had his BP checked in the pharmacy, and it was 142/80 mm Hg. You take his BP today, and it is 138/78 mm Hg. What may be the cause of the elevated systolic BP?
    a. Anxiety
    b. Gender
    c. Age
    d. Systolic hypertension

16. Potential causes of secondary hypertension include all of the following except
    a. increased water intake.
    b. renal artery stenosis.
    c. thyroid disorders.
    d. coarctation of the aorta.

17. When checking the respiratory rate in your patient, it is important not to tell the patient that you are checking his respirations because
    a. you need to check the ratio between pulse and respirations.
    b. the patient may vary the rate or pattern of breathing.
    c. the patient may hold his or her breath while you are counting.
    d. the patient may begin breathing through his or her mouth rather than his or her nose.

18. Select the best method for checking the patients pulse.
    a. Count for 30 seconds and multiply by 2.
    b. Count the pulse for 15 seconds and multiply by 4.
    c. Count the pulse for 10 seconds and multiply by 6.
    d. Count the pulse after you have assessed the contour and amplitude.

19. If the BP cuff is too loose, it will result in
    a. an inaccurate BP reading.
    b. an inaccurate diastolic reading.
    c. an inaccurate systolic reading.
    d. no changes in the BP results.

20. Orthostatic hypertension is
    a. systolic BP drop greater than 5 mm Hg and a diastolic drop of 5 mm Hg.
    b. systolic BP drop greater than 10 mm Hg and a diastolic drop of 10 mm Hg.
    c. systolic BP drop greater than 20 mm Hg and a diastolic drop of 10 mm Hg.
    d. systolic BP drop greater than 20 mm Hg and a diastolic drop of 20 mm Hg.

5 Mental Status

LEARNING OBJECTIVES

After studying Chapter 5 in the textbook and completing this section of the laboratory manual, students should be able to:
1. Identify aspects of an interview that facilitate mental status examination.
2. Describe techniques to assess mental status in the following areas: physical appearance, cognitive abilities, emotional stability, speech, and language skills.
3. Recognize mental status findings that deviate from expected findings.
4. Compare and contrast common conditions affecting mental status.
5. Identify conditions affecting mental status in various age groups.

TEXTBOOK REVIEW

Chapter 5: Mental Status (pp. 64–78)

CHAPTER OVERVIEW

This chapter is designed to help students develop effective techniques to assess mental status. This chapter focuses on mental status evaluation of the individual's overall cognitive state. Additional mental status examination techniques are discussed, and helpful devices related to a mental status examination are reviewed. Finally, this chapter evaluates mental status examination findings in relation to common abnormalities of patients of various populations.

TERMINOLOGY REVIEW

Affect—an emotional response or feeling.

Aging—process of decline in synthesis and metabolism of neurotransmitters.

Analogy—a figure of speech wherein objects or concepts are compared.

Anxiety—a group of disorders with marked apprehension or fear that causes significant interference with personal, social, and occupational functioning.

Aphasia—a speech disorder that can be receptive (understanding language) or expressive (speaking language); it may be indicated by hesitations and other speech rhythm disturbances, omission of syllables or words, word transposition, circumlocutions, and neologisms.

Apraxia—the inability to translate an intention into action that is unrelated to paralysis or lack of comprehension; may indicate a cerebral disorder.

Attention-deficit/hyperactivity disorder (ADHD)—a neurobehavioral problem of impaired attention and hyperactive behavior affecting 5% to 10% of school-age children.

Autism—a pervasive neurodevelopmental disorder of unknown etiology; refers to a wide spectrum of disorders typically developing before 3 years of age more often in boys than girls.

Broca—area associated with speech formation.

Cerebral cortex—the part of the brain that houses the higher mental functions and is responsible for perception and behavior.

Cerebrum—lobe of the brain primarily responsible for mental status.

Cognitive—pertaining to mental processes of memory, judgment, and reasoning; cognitive impairment is characterized by a loss of memory, confusion, and inappropriate affect.

Coherence—a patient's intentions or perceptions should be clearly conveyed to you.

Comprehension—capacity of the mind to understand; demonstrated by an ability to follow simple instructions.

Concussion—an alteration in mental status resulting from a blow to the head or neck.

Cortex—part of the cerebrum responsible for perception and behavior.

Delirium—impaired cognition, consciousness, mood, and behavioral dysfunction of acute onset.

Dementia—a chronic, slowly progressive disorder of failing memory, cognitive impairment, behavioral abnormalities, and personality changes that often begins after age 60 years.

Depression—a mood disorder in which feelings of sadness, loss, anger, or frustration interfere with everyday life for an extended period of time.

Dysarthria—a motor speech disorder defect associated with many conditions of the nervous system such as stroke, inebriation, cerebral palsy, and Parkinson disease.

Dysphonia—a disorder of voice volume, quality, or pitch.

Glasgow Come Scale—a coma scale used to assess the function of the cerebral cortex and brainstem and to quantify consciousness.

Hallucination—a sensory experience not due to external stimulus.

Insults—events in the brain such as trauma, infection, or chemical imbalance can damage brain cells that may result in serious permanent dysfunction in mental status.

Intellectual disability—a developmental, cognitive, or intellectual deficit with accompanying deficits in adaptive behavior, academic performance, adaptive functioning that begins before 18 years of age; previously called mental retardation.

Judgment—the ability to reason.

Limbic—referring to the system that mediates patterns of behavior that determine survival such as mating, aggression, fear, and affection.

Mania—persistently elevated, expansive, euphoric or irritable and agitated mood lasting longer than 1 week; one phase of the bipolar psychiatric disorder.

Mini-Mental State Examination (MMSE)—a brief standardized screening tool used to assess cognitive function and to detect changes over time.

Parietal—referring to the lobe of the brain primarily responsible for processing sensory data.

Schizophrenia—severe persistent, psychotic syndrome that relapses throughout life.

Temporal—referring to the lobe of the brain responsible for perception and the interpretation of sounds.

Wernicke—area of the temporal lobe that permits comprehension of spoken and written language.

APPLICATION TO CLINICAL PRACTICE

Matching

Match each mental status term with its corresponding definition.

Definition	Mental Status Term
_____ 1. Feelings of helplessness	a. Mood lability
_____ 2. Apprehension	b. Anxiety
_____ 3. Excessive happiness	c. Flat affect
_____ 4. Rapid shift of emotions	d. Depression
_____ 5. Lack of emotional response	e. Irritability
_____ 6. Annoyed response to stimulus	f. Euphoria

Clinical Concepts Application

List ways that the following aspects of cognitive abilities might be assessed during examination. For each assessment, briefly describe how a patient's response would be evaluated.

1. Attention

2. Memory

3. Judgment

4. Abstract reasoning

5. Thought processes and content

Clinical Case Study

Mrs. Mildred Cobb, age 78 years, is brought to the geriatric clinic by her son and daughter-in-law. Mrs. Cobb's son tells the examiner that his father passed away 5 months ago, and ever since then, his mother has "gone downhill." Mr. Cobb indicates that his mother is no longer keeping her house clean or cooking appropriate meals. Also, her personal hygiene habits have changed dramatically. She has lost interest in getting her hair done, and she no longer likes to get dressed for the day. Mr. Cobb tells the examiner, "When I suggest a retirement home, she becomes very angry and tells me to mind my own business. I am just worried about Mom, and I want to make sure she is well cared for." During this conversation, Mrs. Cobb sits quietly. She interjects only to say, "I have taken care of you, your brother, and your father. Now, all of a sudden, you think I am helpless and want to lock me away." Mrs. Cobb appears clean, although her hair is matted, and her clothes are badly wrinkled and do not match. Her speech is clear, but her overall affect is very dull. She does not make eye contact with her son or the examiner. A physical examination demonstrates normal bodily functioning consistent with her age group.

1. Which data deviate from normal findings, suggesting altered mental health?

2. What additional questions could the examiner ask to clarify Mrs. Cobb's symptoms?

3. What additional physical examination, if any, should the examiner complete?

4. Mrs. Cobb's symptoms are consistent with what condition affecting mental health?

CRITICAL THINKING

1. How are depression, delirium, and dementia differentiated?

2. What types of changes in mental functioning can be expected in an older adult? Address personality, intellectual function, problem-solving skills, and memory.

CONTENT REVIEW QUESTIONS

Multiple Choice

Circle the correct answer for each of the following questions.

1. A patient's inability to follow simple instructions could indicate which of the following findings?
   a. Dysphonia
   b. Amnesia
   c. Aphasia
   d. Depression

2. A patient scores a 22 out of 40 on an Isaac Set Test to evaluate mental function as a whole. What does this score indicate?
   a. Possible depression
   b. Possible dementia
   c. Need for further evaluation
   d. Normal functioning

3. The examiner asks the patient to complete this statement: "A bird is to air as a fish is to . . . ." This is an example of what type of testing?
   a. Calculation
   b. Analogy
   c. Judgment
   d. Mood and feelings

4. Assume that the patient's response to the examiner in question 4 is "scales." What does this response likely reflect?
   a. Left cerebral hemisphere lesion
   b. Depression
   c. Eating disorder
   d. Aphasia

5. What technique should be used to evaluate the mental status of a patient with head trauma?
   a. MMSE
   b. Perceptual distortion assessment
   c. Glasgow Coma Scale
   d. Functional assessment

6. Which of the following indicates possible cognitive impairment?
   a. Ability to complete personal care without assistance
   b. Suspiciousness or inappropriate affect
   c. Articulate communication
   d. Prudent behavior and calm demeanor

7. A 65-year-old woman is brought to the clinic by family members, who report that they have noticed a change in her mental abilities over the past 2 weeks. Normally, they say, she is independent, intelligent, and very socially oriented. Her medical history is unremarkable except for congestive heart failure, for which she takes digoxin. She has had no major changes in her health. What question would be the most important for the examiner to ask this woman's family?
   a. "Is there a family history of Alzheimer disease?"
   b. "How much alcohol does she drink in an average week?"
   c. "When was her digoxin blood level last checked?"
   d. "Did you know that mental function begins to decline after the age of 60?"

8. A patient who has difficulty writing or drawing is most likely to have which condition?
   a. Cerebral dysfunction
   b. Peripheral neuropathy
   c. Organic brain syndrome
   d. Psychiatric hallucinations
   e. Stupor

9. A mother brings her 18-month-old son to the clinic. She states that the child rarely talks or smiles or makes eye contact. She has also noticed that he does not like to be held. She says his motor development seems to be normal. These symptoms are consistent with what condition?
   a. Dementia
   b. Autistic disorder
   c. ADHD
   d. Delirium

10. A patient with Alzheimer disease classically displays which of the following?
    a. Alternating level of orientation—good during the day but poor at night
    b. Hallucinations and decorticate posturing
    c. Disintegration of personality
    d. Rapid onset of symptoms

6 Growth and Measurement

After studying Chapter 6 in the textbook and completing this section of the laboratory manual, students should be able to:
1. Recognize anatomic and physiologic factors that influence growth.
2. Identify interview methods to gather data pertinent to growth and development.
3. Describe tools and instruments used to assess developmental achievement.
4. Identify expected findings relevant to growth and development throughout the life span.
5. Describe variations in findings that may be considered within normal range.

TEXTBOOK REVIEW

Chapter 6: Growth and Measurement (pp. 79–94)

CHAPTER OVERVIEW

This chapter focuses on the evaluation of an individual's body size and the examination for growth, gestational age, and pubertal development. Physical examination techniques, as well as appropriate tools and instruments used to assess developmental achievement, are evaluated. Also discussed are growth and measurement differences by organ system and special populations. Finally, the chapter examines selected growth and measurement abnormalities and the clinical characteristics discovered during health assessment.

TERMINOLOGY REVIEW

Acromegaly—a rare disease of excessive growth and distorted proportions caused by hypersecretion of growth hormone and insulin-like growth factor after closure of the epiphyses.

Ballard gestational age assessment—an assessment tool that evaluates six physical and six neuromuscular characteristics within 36 hours of birth to establish or confirm the newborn's gestational age.

Body mass index—the most common method used to assess nutritional status and total body fat.

Cushing syndrome—a disorder associated with a prolonged and excessively high exposure to glucocorticoids.

Failure to thrive—falling one or more standard deviations off growth curve pattern below the fifth percentile for weight and height.

Gestational age—an indicator of a newborn's maturity.

Head circumference—a measurement that should be obtained on each visit until a child reaches 2 years of age.

Hydrocephalus—an excess volume of cerebrospinal fluid in the brain leading to an enlarged head circumference or increased intracranial pressure.

Recumbent length—measurement of the length of increase between birth and 24 months of age in the supine position on the measuring device.

Sexual maturity rating—a marker used to determine a child's pubertal development.

Turner syndrome—a genetic disorder in which there is partial or complete absence of the second X chromosome.

Velocity—a parameter of growth calculated by charting changes in height over a time interval.

1. Normal growth and development require the interaction of many hormones. Describe each of the following hormone's activity in the body.
    a. Growth hormone

    b. Growth hormone–releasing hormone (GHRH)

    c. Somatostatin

    d. Insulin-like growth factor 1 (IGF-1)

2. Growth at puberty is dependent on the interaction of hormones. For each of the following hormones, describe the action in the body.
    a. Sex steroids (androgens)

    b. Testosterone

    c. Estrogen

3. What is the role of leptin in growth of the body?

Matching

Match each description with the hormone disorder it represents.

Characteristic	Hormone Disorder
_____ 1. A 16-year-old female with absence of sexual development; also has short stature and increased carrying angle of the elbows	a. Acromegaly
	b. Adolescence
_____ 2. Woman with hyperpigmentation to the skin, round face, and fat accumulation in the lower posterior cervical area	c. Cushing syndrome
_____ 3. A 5-year-old girl with pubertal changes	d. Hydrocephalus
_____ 4. Child with pronounced head enlargement and increased intracranial pressure	e. Precocious puberty
_____ 5. Half of an individual's ideal weight gained during this period	f. Turner syndrome
_____ 6. A 60-year-old man with exaggerated facial features and massive hands	

CONTENT REVIEW QUESTIONS

Multiple Choice

Circle the correct answer for each of the following questions.

1. A patient's frame size can be estimated by
   a. dividing the height by the weight.
   b. dividing the height by half the weight.
   c. measuring the head circumference.
   d. measuring the elbow breadth.

2. A 38-year-old woman is 5 feet, 7 inches tall; weighs 163 pounds; and has an elbow breadth of 6.9 cm. Based on these measurements, the examiner estimates her frame size as
   a. extra small.
   b. small.
   c. medium.
   d. large.

3. The body mass index of the patient in question 2 would be
   a. 21.
   b. 25.5.
   c. 27.
   d. 29.5.

4. Brain growth is completed by
   a. 1 year of age.
   b. 2 years of age.
   c. 3 years of age.
   d. 7 years of age.

5. A child has an arm span that measures greater than his height. This finding is consistent with what condition?
   a. Turner syndrome
   b. Marfan syndrome
   c. Acromegaly
   d. Failure to thrive

6. Growth at puberty is dependent on the interaction of which of the following?
   a. IGF-1 and sex steroids
   b. luteinizing hormone [LH] and follicle-stimulating hormone [FSH]
   c. GHRH and IGF-1
   d. Estrogen and testosterone

7. To accurately assess height velocity, the examiner must measure a child's height at
   a. 6-month intervals.
   b. about 9-month intervals.
   c. 12-month intervals.
   d. 14-month intervals.

8. A pregnant patient has a prepregnancy body mass index of 22.4. The examiner expects this patient's weight gain during pregnancy to fall into which weight range?
   a. Less than 20 pounds
   b. 20 to 26 pounds
   c. 25 to 35 pounds
   d. 40 to 50 pounds

9. The beginning of adolescence is marked by the
   a. 12th birthday.
   b. development of selfish, impatient behavioral traits.
   c. development of a conscience and a sense of morality.
   d. onset of puberty.

10. To assess and monitor growth, the examiner makes routine measurements of an infant's weight, height/length, and which of the following?
   a. Head circumference
   b. Hip-to-toe length
   c. Forearm length
   d. Chest circumference

11. A 4-month-old infant is brought to the clinic. At birth, the baby weighed 6 pounds 8 ounces. If the baby is gaining weight at a desired rate, the examiner should expect the baby to now weigh
   a. 8 pounds.
   b. 9.5 pounds.
   c. 12 pounds.
   d. 15 pounds.

12. Which hormone has a key role in regulating body fat mass and is thought to be a trigger for puberty?
   a. Leptin
   b. Androgens
   c. Estrogen
   d. Growth hormone

7 Nutrition

LEARNING OBJECTIVES

After studying Chapter 7 in the textbook and completing this section of the laboratory manual, students should be able to:
1. Describe interview techniques used to obtain a nutritional history.
2. Identify components of a nutritional examination.
3. Analyze data gained from a nutritional examination.
4. Identify common nutritional conditions.
5. List macronutrients and micronutrients required by the body.

TEXTBOOK REVIEW

Chapter 7: Nutrition (pp. 95–113)

CHAPTER OVERVIEW

This chapter examines interview techniques effective in gathering information for a nutritional assessment. In addition, this chapter reviews the use of nutrients for growth, development, and maintenance of health. Finally, this chapter analyzes significant nutritional abnormalities, their effect on the health status of the patient, and their effect on results in physical examination findings.

TERMINOLOGY REVIEW

Anemia—a lower-than-normal number of circulating red blood cells.
Anorexia nervosa—a psychiatric disease characterized by low body weight and body image distortion.
Bulimia—eating disorder characterized by binge eating.
Carbohydrates—the body's main source of energy, found mostly in plants and in milk.
Cheilosis—a clinical finding caused by pyridoxine and iron deficiency.
Cholesterol—a substance associated with coronary heart disease and recommended intake at less than 200 mg/day.
Essential amino acids—nine amino acids are considered essential; a type of amino acid that cannot be synthesized in the body.
Fat—the body's main source of linoleic acid and alpha-linolenic acid.
Glycogen—a stored form of carbohydrates.
Macronutrients—nutrients required by the body in large amounts (carbohydrates, fats, and proteins).
Micronutrients—nutrients required and stored by the body in small amounts.
Midarm muscle circumference—a sensitive index of protein reserves.
Nutrition—the science of food as it relates to promoting optimal health and preventing chronic disease.
Obesity—excessive proportion of total body fat.
Pica—nonnutritive eating.
Protein—nutrient made up of amino acids.
Resting energy expenditure—the largest proportion of total energy expenditure by the body.
Thermogenesis—metabolic rate increases in response to food intake.
Water—the nutrient most vital to the body.

Clinical Case Study 1

The following patients have appointments at the medical clinic:
  15-year-old male weighing 110 pounds
  25-year-old female weighing 142 pounds
  32-year-old female weighing 200 pounds
  62-year-old male weighing 168 pounds

1. Which of these patients would you guess has the highest resting energy expenditure? Calculate the resting energy expenditure based on age and body weight for the four patients. (Refer to Table 7-1 on p. 97 in the textbook for assistance.)

   15-year-old male weighing 110 pounds: _____ kcal/day

   25-year-old female weighing 142 pounds: _____ kcal/day

   32-year-old female weighing 200 pounds: _____ kcal/day

   62-year-old male weighing 168 pounds: _____ kcal/day

Case Study 2

Jack is a 43-year-old man who complains of a loss of energy, loss of appetite, and loss of weight. He states that he used to maintain a steady weight of 172 pounds but that over the past 9 months he has gradually lost weight. Jack is 5 feet, 9 inches tall and currently weighs 142 pounds. He has a midarm muscle circumference of 255 mm.

1. Calculate Jack's desirable weight based on height and weight.

   Desirable body weight: _____

2. Calculate Jack's percentage of desirable body weight.

   Percent of desirable body weight: _____

3. Calculate Jack's percentage of his usual body weight.

   Percent of usual body weight: _____

4. What percentage of weight change has Jack experienced with this illness?

   Percent of weight change: _____

5. Calculate Jack's current body mass index (BMI). (Refer to Box 7-4 on p. 100 in the textbook for help.)

   Current BMI: _____

6. What was his previous BMI (before his weight loss)?

   Previous BMI: _____

7. In what percentile would Jack be categorized based on his midarm muscle circumference?

8. What conclusions can you make about Jack based on your calculations above?

Personal Food Record

1. Complete a 24-hour food recall, listing all foods, beverages, and snacks eaten during the past 24 hours.

Personal Food Assessment

Visit the ChooseMyPlate.gov website to create a Daily Food Plan based on your age, gender, weight, height, and physical activity.

Personal Analysis of Nutritional Needs

1. Analyze the data you have gathered during your personal food record and personal food assessment above. Compare your results with the suggested daily servings from the ChooseMyPlate.gov website.

A One-Day (24-Hour) Record of Food Intake

NAME _____   DATE OF RECORD _____

BREAKFAST   Time Eaten _____

Food/Beverage	Type and/or Method of Preparation (List Ingredients)	Amount
MILK		
FRUIT fresh, canned, sweetened, etc.		
CEREAL _____ with milk _____ with sugar _____ other	Brand _____	
BREAD _____ margarine/butter _____ mayonnaise _____ other	White _____ Brown _____	
EGGS		
MEAT or OTHER PROTEIN		
BEVERAGE _____ with milk _____ with sugar _____ other		
OTHER FOODS		

Did you eat a mid-morning snack?   Yes _____   No _____   If yes, time? _____
(List foods and beverages eaten.)

_____

_____

NOON MEAL   Time Eaten _____

Food/Beverage	Type and/or Method of Preparation (List Ingredients)	Amount
SOUP		
BREAD _____ margarine/butter _____ mayonnaise _____ other	White _____ Brown _____	
_____ MEAT _____ EGG _____ FISH _____ CHEESE		
VEGETABLES _____ cooked _____ raw _____ topping/seasoning (butter, white sauce, cheese sauce, etc.)		
SALAD _____ dressing (brand, etc.)		
FRUIT fresh, canned, sweetened, etc.		
MILK		
BEVERAGE _____ with milk _____ with sugar _____ other		
DESSERT		
OTHER FOODS		

Did you eat an afternoon snack? Yes _____   No _____   If yes, time? _____
(List foods and beverages eaten.)

_____

_____

EVENING MEAL   Time Eaten _____

Food/Beverage	Type and/or Method of Preparation (List Ingredients)	Amount
MAIN DISH _____ meat _____ cheese _____ poultry _____ other protein _____ pasta _____ rice		
VEGETABLES _____ cooked _____ raw _____ topping/seasoning (butter, white sauce, cheese sauce, etc.)		
SALAD _____ dressing (brand, etc.)		
BREAD _____ margarine/butter _____ mayonnaise _____ other	White _____ Brown _____	
FRUIT fresh, canned, sweetened, etc.		
MILK		
BEVERAGE _____ with milk _____ with sugar _____ other		
DESSERT		
OTHER FOODS		

Did you eat an evening snack? Yes _____   No _____   If yes, time? _____
(List foods and beverages eaten.)

_____

_____

Modified from Burke B: The dietary history as a tool in research, *J Am Dietic Assoc* 23:1044–1046, 1947.

Match the sign or symptom with the vitamin deficiency

Sign or Symptom	Vitamin Deficiency
_____ 1. Alopecia	a. Niacin
_____ 2. Corneal vascularization	b. Protein
_____ 3. Atopic dermatitis	c. Riboflavin
_____ 4. Edema	d. Pyridoxine
_____ 5. Arthralgia	e. Zinc
_____ 6. Stomatitis	f. Vitamin C

CRITICAL THINKING

1. Macronutrients include carbohydrates, protein, and fats. Describe each of these nutrients below.
   a. Carbohydrates

   b. Protein

   c. Fats

2. Micronutrients are required and stored in very small quantities by the body. Describe the general function of micronutrients such as vitamins, minerals, and electrolytes and explain how they differ from the macronutrients.

3. Which micronutrients can be synthesized by the body?

Multiple Choice

Circle the correct answer for each of the following questions.

1. During an interview, the patient reports that she frequently has sores at the corners of her mouth. What type of nutritional deficiency should be considered?
   a. Vitamin E
   b. Protein
   c. B vitamins
   d. Fatty acid

2. An adolescent-aged patient has a low-density lipoprotein (LDL) level drawn. A diagnosis of hyperlipidemia would be made only if the patient's LDL level is above
   a. 100 mg/dL.
   b. 120 mg/dL.
   c. 130 mg/dL.
   d. 160 mg/dL.

3. A dietary assessment is performed by
   a. comparing established eating habits with the recommended dietary allowances.
   b. asking the patient to fill out a food pyramid.
   c. comparing the recommended dietary allowances to the U.S. Department of Agriculture MyPyramid.
   d. asking the patient to do a 24-hour dietary recall.

4. Ideally, for an adult, the percentage of total calories coming from fat should be limited to
   a. 10%.
   b. 30%.
   c. 40%.
   d. 50%.

5. Which of the following laboratory tests is an indicator for protein status of a patient?
   a. Albumin
   b. Blood urea nitrogen and creatinine
   c. Electrolytes
   d. Complete blood count

6. A patient's hair is very dull and can be easily plucked. The patient is also very thin and appears to have significant muscle wasting. Based on these findings, what other objective data might the examiner anticipate?
   a. Thyroid enlargement
   b. Hepatomegaly
   c. Spongy bleeding gums
   d. Ecchymoses and petechiae

7. Healthy eating guidelines recommend how many servings of the milk, yogurt, and cheese group each day for an adult male?
   a. One
   b. Two
   c. Three
   d. Five

8. MyPyramid recommends 6 to 11 servings from the bread, cereal, and grain products group. Which of the following represents one serving from that group?
   a. 1 cup of cooked rice
   b. 6 soda crackers
   c. 1 hamburger bun
   d. 1 slice of bread

9. It is difficult to calculate the exact energy expenditure of a given activity for a specific patient because of individual variables such as
   a. height.
   b. type of fat cells.
   c. muscle mass.
   d. dietary intake.

10. A mother is concerned that her 16-year-old son is not eating enough protein. The young man is 5 feet, 5 inches tall and weighs 125 pounds. Referring to Appendix E on the Evolve website, what is the recommended amount of protein intake?
    a. 45 g/day
    b. 51 g/day
    c. 110 g/day
    d. 112 g/day

11. Physical findings associated with protein deficiency include muscle wasting, dull hair, and
    a. a magenta tongue.
    b. follicular hyperkeratosis.
    c. edema to the extremities.
    d. Bitot spots.

12. Females from which of the following groups are at the highest risk for eating disorders?
    a. Honor roll students who excel in math and English
    b. Teenagers who enjoy eating pizza with friends on the weekend
    c. Children from low-income families
    d. College-age students who are perfectionists

13. Which of the following laboratory values rules out the likelihood that a patient has a vitamin B_{12} deficiency?
    a. Serum iron of 42 mcg/dL
    b. Transferrin saturation of 30%
    c. Hemoglobin level of 14 g/dL
    d. Hematocrit level of 35%

14. During an examination, a patient tells the examiner she would like to lose weight. She is 5 feet, 7 inches tall and weighs 186 pounds. Using a quick estimate for energy needs, how many kcal/kg would be appropriate for weight loss for this patient?
    a. 20 kcal/kg
    b. 25 kcal/kg
    c. 30 kcal/kg
    d. 35 kcal/kg

15. The target kcal/day for the patient in question 15 would be
    a. 1642 kcal/day.
    b. 1994 kcal/day.
    c. 2112 kcal/day.
    d. 2412 kcal/day.

16. It is known that a person's metabolic rate increases after eating. How much of an increase occurs in the total energy expenditure of the body?
    a. 5%
    b. 7%
    c. 10%
    d. 12%

17. To assess an older patient's ability to consume foods, the examiner should
    a. examine the back, arms, and shoulders for evidence of muscle wasting.
    b. examine the skin for dryness or elasticity.
    c. assess the abdomen for fullness, distention, and bowel sounds.
    d. assess the oral cavity for the condition of the teeth and presence of lesions.

18. A waist-to-hip circumference ratio greater than 0.9 in men and 0.8 in women indicates which of the following?
    a. A healthy nutritional status
    b. A low percentage of body fat
    c. A large body frame
    d. An increased risk for disease

8 | Skin, Hair, and Nails

LEARNING OBJECTIVES

After studying Chapter 8 in the textbook and completing this section of the laboratory manual, students should be able to:

1. Conduct a history related to skin, hair, and nails.
2. Discuss examination techniques for skin, hair, and nails.
3. Identify normal age and condition variations to the skin, hair, and nails.
4. Recognize findings that deviate from expected results.
5. Relate symptoms or clinical findings to common pathologic conditions.

TEXTBOOK REVIEW

Chapter 8: Skin, Hair, and Nails (pp. 114–165)

CHAPTER OVERVIEW

This chapter reviews the anatomy and physiology of the skin, hair, and nails, including specific findings for special populations such as older adults, infants, and children. The key elements of a related history are reviewed to assist the learner in focusing the physical examination. Finally, the common abnormalities of the skin, hair, and nails as related to the health and physical assessment of the patient are described.

TERMINOLOGY REVIEW

Acrocyanosis—a bluish discoloration of the hands and feet may be present at birth and may persist for several days or longer if the newborn is kept in cool ambient temperatures.

Alopecia—hair loss.

Alopecia areata—sudden, rapid, patchy loss of hair, usually from the scalp or face.

Annular—round, active margins with central clearing.

Apocrine glands—specialized structures found only in the axillae, nipples, areolae, anogenital area, eyelids, and external ears.

Cellular stratum—one of the major layers in the epidermis, where keratin cells are synthesized.

Cellulitis—a diffuse, acute infection of the skin and subcutaneous tissue.

Chloasma—occurs in pregnant women and is found on the forehead, cheeks, bridge of the nose, and chin; it is blotchy and symmetrical.

Confluent—referring to lesions that run together.

Cutis marmorata—a mottled appearance of the body and extremities of the skin of a newborn when exposed to decreased temperatures.

Dermatomal—referring to a lesion that follows a nerve or segment of the body.

Dermis—richly vascular connective tissue layer of the skin that supports and separates the epidermis from the cutaneous adipose tissue.

Ecchymosis—a discoloration produced by injury.

Eccrine glands—glands that open directly to the skin surface and are found throughout the body except in the lip margins, eardrums, nail beds, inner surface of the prepuce, and glans penis.

Eczematous dermatitis—the most common inflammatory skin disorder; several forms exist, including irritant contact dermatitis, allergic contact dermatitis, and atopic dermatitis.

Epidermis—the outer portion of skin, consists of two layers.

Erythema toxicum—a pink papular rash with vesicles superimposed on thorax, back, buttocks, and abdomen in newborns about 36 hours after birth.

Folliculitis—inflammation and infection of the hair follicle and surrounding dermis.

Furuncle—a deep-seated infection of the pilosebaceous unit.

Generalized—widely distributed or present in several areas simultaneously.

Herpes simplex—infection caused by the herpes simplex virus.

Herpes zoster—infection cause by the varicella zoster virus.

Hypodermis—layer of skin that connects the dermis to the underlying organs that consists of loose connective tissue filled with fatty cells.

Keloid—irregular-shaped, elevated, progressively enlarging hypertrophied scar tissue.

Keratin—waterproofing protein found in the stratum corneum.

Lanugo—fine, silky hair of newborns found on the shoulders and back.

Melanin—synthesized in the stratum germinativum by melanocytes and is the pigment that gives skin its color.

Mongolian spots—irregular areas of deep blue pigmentation on the sacral and gluteal regions of a newborn; most predominantly occurs in people of African, Native American, Asian, or Latin descent.

Morbilliform—refers to maculopapular lesions that become confluent on the face and body.

Nails—epidermal cells converted to hard plates of keratin.

Nevus—a mole that varies in size and degree of pigmentation.

Papillae—loops of capillaries that supply nourishment for hair follicles.

Petechiae—tiny, flat, purple or red spots on the skin surface, resulting from minute hemorrhages within the dermal layer smaller than 0.5 cm in diameter.

Pityriasis rosea—self-limiting inflammation of unknown cause.

Plaque—a type of skin lesion common in patients with psoriasis.

Psoriasis—a chronic and recurrent disease of keratin synthesis.

Pruritic urticarial papules and plaque of pregnancy—a benign dermatosis that usually arises late in the third trimester of a first pregnancy.

Reticulate—referring to a lesion with a netlike or lacy appearance.

Rosacea—a chronic inflammatory skin disorder.

Salmon patches (stork bites)—flat, deep pink localized areas usually seen on the mid-forehead, eyelids, upper lip, and back of neck in a newborn.

Sebum—a lipid substance that keeps skin and hair from drying out.

Serpiginous—referring to lesions that appear to occur in a wavy line.

Stellate—referring to a star-shaped lesion.

Stratum corneum—the outermost layer of the dermis, which protects the body against environmental stressors and water loss.

Stratum lucidum—layer of dermis found in thicker skin on the palms and soles.

Telangiectasis—permanently dilated, small blood vessels consisting of venules, capillaries, or arterioles.

Terminal hair—course, longer, thicker, and usually pigmented hair.

Tinea—a group of noncandidal fungal infections that involve the stratum corneum, nails, and hair.

Vellus hair—short, fine hair that is nonpigmented.

Vernix caseosa—a mixture of sebum and cornified epidermis that covers the infant's body at birth.

Vesicle—a fluid-filled and elevated, but superficial, skin lesion.

Wood's lamp—type of lamp used to evaluate epidermal hypopigmented or hyperpigmented lesion and to distinguish the fluorescing skin lesions.

APPLICATION TO CLINICAL PRACTICE

Anatomy Review

Identify structures on the diagram of the nail by writing the correct term in the blank next to the corresponding letter.

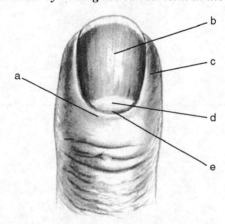

a. _____

b. _____

c. _____

d. _____

e. _____

Clinical Concepts Application

Identify the type of secondary lesion shown in each illustration below. For each type of lesion, give one or more common examples.

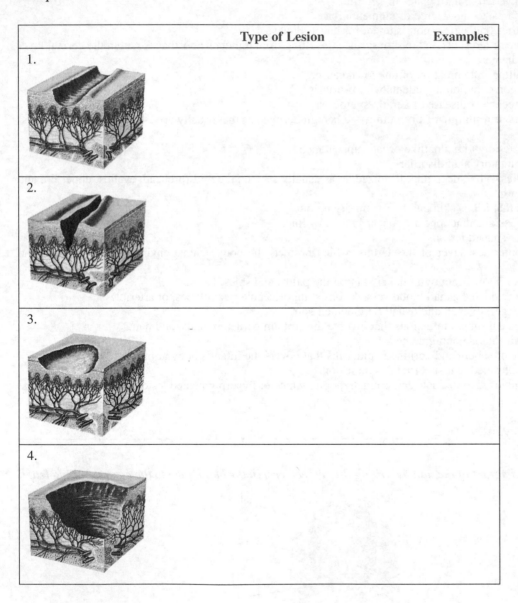

	Type of Lesion	Examples
1.		
2.		
3.		
4.		

Matching 1

Match each type of lesion with its corresponding description or the condition with which the lesion is commonly associated.

Description or Associated Condition	Type of Lesion
_____ 1. Chickenpox	a. Papule
_____ 2. Insect bite	b. Macule
_____ 3. Impetigo	c. Vesicle
_____ 4. Chronic dermatitis	d. Nodule
_____ 5. Lipoma	e. Pustule
_____ 6. Blister	f. Patch
_____ 7. Wart	g. Lichenification
_____ 8. Port wine stain	h. Wheal
_____ 9. Petechiae	i. Bulla

Matching 2

Match the dermatologic finding with its appropriate description.

Dermatologic Finding	Description
_____ 1. Palmar erythema	a. Contagious staphylococcal or streptococcal infection of the epidermis
_____ 2. Sebaceous hyperplasia	b. Yellowish, flattened papules with central depression
_____ 3. Cystic acne	c. Inflammatory lesions; nodules, and comedones larger than 5 mm
_____ 4. Impetigo	d. Diffuse redness over palmar surface during pregnancy

Matching 3

Match each part of the skin anatomy with the area in which it is found. (Note: Letters will be used more than once.)

Skin Anatomy	Area Found
_____ 1. Stratum corneum	a. Epidermis
_____ 2. Autonomic motor nerves	b. Dermis
_____ 3. Cellular stratum	c. Hypodermis
_____ 4. Basement membrane	
_____ 5. Reticulum fibers	
_____ 6. Subcutaneous layer	
_____ 7. Stratum germinativum	
_____ 8. Layer that generates heat	

Clinical Case Study

Mr. John Tate is a 74-year-old man who comes to the clinic for a "routine checkup." Listed below are data collected by the examiner on the patient's skin, hair, and nails.

INTERVIEW DATA

Mr. Tate denies any specific complaints except that he has some nonpainful sores on his legs that "don't seem to want to heal."

EXAMINATION DATA

Hair distribution: Full head of hair that is coarse and thinning. No areas of balding noted. Hair color is gray.

Overall appearance of skin: Skin is pale pink, thin, and dry with flaking and tenting present.

Face and neck: Pigmented, raised, warty lesions (seborrheic keratosis) noted on face. Three cutaneous tags noted on neck. Several senile lentigines lesions noted on neck and face.

Chest and abdomen: 1–mm, tiny, bright red round papules (cherry angiomas) noted on chest. Angular surgical scar noted in right upper abdomen.

Extremities: Legs and ankles have areas of erythematous, scaling, and weeping patches. Legs slightly edematous. No hair growth noted on legs. Upper arms: Skin very thin and dry; several senile lentigines lesions noted on arms bilaterally.

Nails: Nails are yellowish and thick but well trimmed.

1. What data deviate from normal findings, suggesting a need for further investigation?

2. What additional questions could be asked by the examiner to clarify symptoms?

3. What additional examination data should be assessed?

4. What type of problem(s) do you think the patient may have?

CRITICAL THINKING

1. Mr. Mason is a 72-year-old man who presents to the clinic with a lesion on his cheek. He says it has been there for years, but his wife has been nagging him to "get it checked out in case it is cancer." After examination, you determine the lesion is a benign mole. However, you tell Mr. Mason to "keep an eye on it." What warning signs would you discuss with him?

2. Mrs. Tran brings her 3-year-old child to the pediatric clinic, informing the examiner that the child is "red all over and cries frequently." The examiner notes a rash on the child's skin. What specific characteristics should be noted when examining and documenting a skin lesion?

CONTENT REVIEW QUESTIONS

Multiple Choice
Circle the correct answer for each of the following questions.

1. Milia are an expected finding in which age group?
   a. Newborns
   b. Young children
   c. Adolescents
   d. Older adults

2. An older patient asks the examiner, "Is this spot on my chin a cancer?" Which of the following would indicate a need for further medical investigation?
   a. Reddish brown color of the lesion
   b. Presence on his chin for 20 years
   c. Bleeds easily when it is touched
   d. Slightly raised and circumscribed

3. A 6-year-old girl has freckles over her nose and cheeks. Freckles are a type of
   a. macule.
   b. papule.
   c. nodule.
   d. petechiae.

4. The examiner suspects that a dark-skinned patient is hypoxic. To assess for the presence of cyanosis, the examiner should
   a. inspect the skin for a deeper tone of brown or black.
   b. inspect for an ashen-gray color, especially in the mucous membranes.
   c. palpate the skin for changes in moisture and texture.
   d. palpate the skin for changes in skin texture.

5. Why do some infants develop a yellowish skin tone on the third or fourth day of life?
   a. Increased formation of subcutaneous tissue causes a yellow hue.
   b. Capillaries broken during the birth process turn the skin yellow as bruises heal.
   c. Yellowish color results from increased fat metabolism and heat production.
   d. Red blood cells that hemolyze after birth may cause a yellow skin hue.

6. An adolescent patient asks the examiner why teens have more problems with acne than children. Which of the following would be an appropriate response?
   a. "Children have better hygiene habits than adolescents because of parental guidance."
   b. "Adolescents have reduced blood flow to the epidermal layer of the skin, making them more susceptible to infections."
   c. "At puberty, adolescents begin to secrete more oil from their sebaceous glands."
   d. "Children have very little skin mass, which prevents development of acne."

7. Chloasma is an expected finding in which of the following?
   a. Newborns
   b. Adolescents
   c. Pregnant women
   d. Older adults

8. While examining the skin of an 87-year-old woman, the examiner observes significant tenting. Which of the following age-associated changes best explains this finding?
   a. Small skin tags form on the neck and back.
   b. The skin becomes thin and takes on a parchment-like appearance.
   c. The skin becomes dry with significant flaking.
   d. There is loss of adipose tissue and loss of elasticity.

9. When assessing for the presence of clubbing, the examiner specifically examines the
   a. width of the nail base.
   b. angle of the nail base.
   c. thickness of the nail.
   d. color of the nail.

10. Which type of lesion sometimes grows out of an already-present nevus?
    a. Malignant melanoma
    b. Squamous cell carcinoma
    c. Basal cell carcinoma
    d. Kaposi sarcoma

11. In young and school-age children, the most common skin lesions are caused by
    a. communicable disease and bacterial infection.
    b. changes in skin color and skin tone, which accompany puberty.
    c. maturation of melanocytes, causing changes in skin color.
    d. skin inflammation from sebaceous gland activity.

12. The examiner notes a large blue-black spot on the buttock of a 4-week-old black neonate. The mother states that the infant was born with it. The examiner should recognize that this
    a. is a common finding.
    b. may indicate child abuse.
    c. is related to birth trauma.
    d. suggests a congenital defect.

13. Which of the following may be associated with neurofibromatosis or pulmonary stenosis?
    a. Café au lait spots
    b. Nevus vasculosus
    c. Port-wine limb stain
    d. Spider angioma

14. Which lesion is an expected finding on the skin of healthy older adults?
    a. Acne vulgaris
    b. Cherry angioma
    c. Miliaria
    d. Trichotillomania

15. When palpating skin surfaces for temperature, the examiner should use the
    a. palmar aspect of the hand.
    b. fingertips of the dominant hand.
    c. dorsal aspect of the hands or fingers.
    d. ulnar surface of the hand.

16. Hyperkeratosis is noted on a patient's palms and soles. The examiner recognizes that this
    a. may be a sign of a systemic disorder.
    b. may be an indication of a congenital heart defect.
    c. is common among individuals with down syndrome.
    d. is considered a normal finding.

17. A patient with diabetes presents to the clinic complaining of an infected foot. Upon removing the patient's sock, the examiner notes an odor that resembles rotting apples. This finding is consistent with what type of infection?
    a. *Pseudomonas aeruginosa*
    b. Peritonitis
    c. Aerobic organism
    d. *Clostridium perfringens*

18. Which finding is consistent with a physical abuse injury in a toddler?
    a. Burn to the skin with a splash pattern
    b. Bruising of the skin over soft tissue
    c. Bruising of the skin over a bony prominence
    d. Café au lait patches

19. Which of the following techniques helps the examiner determine whether a palpable skin mass is filled with fluid?
    a. Using a Wood's lamp
    b. Palpating
    c. Transilluminating
    d. Noting the odor of the lesion

20. Which of the following findings suggests that a patient has a fungal infection of the nail beds?
    a. The nail bed is wide and thick.
    b. The nail plate has a central depression, causing a spoon appearance.
    c. Superficial white spots are present in the nail plate.
    d. The nail plate is yellow and crumbling.

9 Lymphatic System

LEARNING OBJECTIVES

After studying Chapter 9 in the textbook and completing this section of the laboratory manual, students should be able to:

1. Conduct a history related to the lymphatic system.
2. Examine techniques for physical examination of the lymphatic system.
3. Identify normal age and condition variations to the lymphatic system.
4. Differentiate normal findings from abnormal findings.
5. Analyze symptoms or clinical findings and relate findings to common pathologic conditions.

TEXTBOOK REVIEW

Chapter 9: Lymphatic System (pp. 166–183)

CHAPTER OVERVIEW

This chapter discusses the anatomy and physiology of the lymphatic system and reviews differentiation for age-specific characteristics. The health history is analyzed, including the components of the History of Present Illness, Personal Medical History, and Family History, specifically in regard to the lymphatic system. The examination techniques of inspection and palpation are discussed relative to the lymphatic system. Finally, common abnormalities of the lymphatic system are analyzed and correlated to common pathologic conditions.

TERMINOLOGY REVIEW

Acute lymphangitis—inflammation of one or more lymphatic vessels.

Acute suppurative lymphadenitis—infection and inflammation of a lymph node; may affect a single node or localized group of nodes.

AIDS—acquired immunodeficiency syndrome; initial symptoms include lymphadenopathy, fatigue, fever, arthralgias, and weight loss.

Epstein-Barr virus mononucleosis—infectious mononucleosis; marked by firm, discrete, tender lymph nodes of anterior and posterior cervical chains and the submandibular lymph nodes.

Fluctuant—wavelike motion that is felt when the node is palpated.

Herpes simplex—a group of acute infections caused by human herpes virus 1 or human herpes virus 2; marked by enlargement of anterior cervical and submandibular nodes.

Hodgkin disease—a malignant lymphoma marked by asymmetric enlargement of the cervical lymph nodes often in the posterior triangle, which are rubbery and nonpainful.

Human immunodeficiency virus (HIV)—characterized by the dysfunction of cell-mediated immunity, HIV seropositivity.

Latex allergy type 1 reaction—true allergic reaction caused by protein antibodies (IgE antibodies) that form as a result of interaction between a foreign protein and the body's immune system.

Lymphadenopathy—enlarged lymph nodes.

Lymphangitis—inflammation of the lymphatics that drain an area of infection; tender erythematous streaks extend proximally from the infected area; regional nodes may also be tender.

Lymphangioma—a congenital malformation of dilated lymphatics.

Lymphatic filariasis—massive accumulation of lymphedema throughout the body; commonly called elephantiasis; most common cause of secondary lymphedema worldwide.

Lymphedema—edematous swelling caused by excessive accumulation of lymph fluid in tissues caused by inadequate lymph drainage.

Matted—group of nodes that feel connected and seem to move as a unit.

Non-Hodgkin lymphoma—a malignant neoplasm of the lymphatic system and the reticuloendothelial tissues; most often in lymph nodes in the chest, neck, abdomen, tonsils, and skin.

Serum sickness (type III hypersensitivity reaction)—an immune complex disease; mediated by tissue deposition of circulating immune complexes.

Shotty nodes—small nontender nodes that feel like BBs or buckshot under the skin.

Toxoplasmosis—a parasitic zoonosis caused by the parasite *Toxoplasma gondii;* marked by a single, chronically enlarged, nontender lymph node in the posterior cervical chain.

APPLICATION TO CLINICAL PRACTICE

Anatomy Review

On the illustration below, complete the activities as instructed.

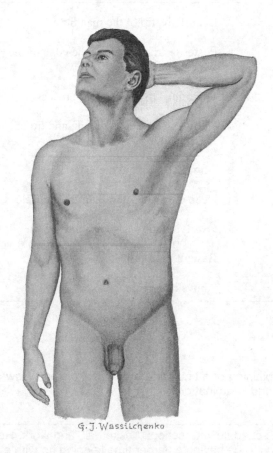

G.J.Wassilchenko

1. Mark the palpable lymph nodes in various regions.

2. Label the various regions of the lymph nodes that you have marked.

3. Indicate with numbers (1 to 6) the order in which you would palpate the head for lymph node examination.

Matching

Match each lymph node with its corresponding location.

Lymph Node	Location
_____ 1. Preauricular	a. Behind the tip of the mandible
_____ 2. Postauricular	b. Posterior triangle along the edge of the trapezius muscle
_____ 3. Occipital	c. Superficial to the mastoid process
_____ 4. Submental	
_____ 5. Submandibular	d. Halfway between the angle and tip of the mandible
_____ 6. Superficial cervical	e. Above and behind the clavicle
_____ 7. Deep cervical	f. Deep under the sternomastoid muscle
_____ 8. Posterior cervical	g. Overlying the sternomastoid muscle
_____ 9. Supraclavicular	h. Base of the skull
	i. Above and behind the ear

Clinical Case Study

Mario is a 16-year-old male complaining of fatigue and weakness. Listed below are data collected by the nurse during an interview and examination.

INTERVIEW DATA

Mario indicates he keeps a busy schedule with school, basketball, and work. He has always been a good student, but now he seems to be having a harder time keeping up with everything. He feels he is beginning to let his family and friends down because fatigue and weakness are interfering with his performance at school and on the basketball court. Mario does not want to quit his job because he is saving for college. When asked about other symptoms, he denies changes in appetite or abdominal problems but reports that he thinks he sometimes has a fever.

EXAMINATION DATA

General survey: Alert, thin male. Height, 5 feet, 7 inches. Weight, 140 pounds.

Skin: Pink color. No evidence of bruising. No skin discoloration.

Head and neck: Enlarged and firm cervical lymph nodes. Supraclavicular nodes also palpable.

Thorax: Respirations even and unlabored, clear to auscultation. Heart rate and rhythm regular.

Abdomen: Bowel sounds auscultated. Abdomen soft, nontender, and nondistended.

Musculoskeletal: Moves all extremities; symmetrical. Moves joints without tenderness.

1. What data deviate from normal findings, suggesting a need for further investigation?

2. What additional questions could be asked by the examiner to clarify symptoms?

3. What additional examination data should be assessed?

4. What type of problem(s) do you think the patient may have?

CRITICAL THINKING

1. How does the lymph system examination of an infant or young child differ from that used for an adult and an older adult? Indicate how findings change with aging.

CONTENT REVIEW QUESTIONS

Multiple Choice
Circle the correct answer for each of the following questions.

1. During an examination, which of the following questions would be most appropriate for the examiner to ask a patient to elicit information about the lymph system?
   a. "Are you aware of any lumps?"
   b. "Have you had a change in appetite?"
   c. "Do your lymph nodes hurt?"
   d. "Where are your largest lymph nodes?"

2. While palpating lymph nodes on an adult, the examiner should remember that
   a. tubercular nodes are hot and firm to the touch.
   b. nodes that are fixed and palpable are a normal finding.
   c. heavy pressure is required to locate and identify nodes.
   d. easily palpable nodes are generally not found in healthy adults.

3. In comparison with those of a young adult, the lymph nodes of an older adult will be
   a. large and soft.
   b. small and fatty.
   c. hard and irregular.
   d. large and hard.

4. A 19-year-old man has a severe infection involving the fifth digit of his right hand. Where should the examiner expect to palpate enlarged and tender lymph nodes?
   a. Radial aspect of the wrist
   b. Palmar aspect of the hand
   c. Medial condyle of the humerus
   d. Preauricular nodes

5. Which of the following examination findings is cause for concern in an adult?
   a. A palpable lymph node moves under the examiner's fingers.
   b. A palpable lymph node is fixed in its setting.
   c. A palpable lymph node is approximately 3 mm in size.
   d. The lymph node is not palpable.

6. The most common causes of acute suppurative lymphadenitis are which organisms?
   a. *Pseudomonas* and *Clostridium* spp.
   b. *Streptococcus* and *Staphylococcus* spp.
   c. *Candida* and *Chlamydia* spp.
   d. *Aspergillus* and *Escherichia* spp.

7. The examiner typically assesses the lymph system using which of the following methods?
   a. Assess the entire lymph system as a unit, exploring all accessible nodes.
   b. Assess both the superficial and deep nodes using palpation and a Doppler study.
   c. Assess the lymph system region by region as each body system is assessed.
   d. Assess the lymph nodes only when the patient's history suggests a need to do so.

8. A 2-month-old infant is brought to the clinic for immunizations. The examiner palpates enlarged inguinal nodes. What additional finding might explain the enlarged nodes?
   a. The mother reports that the infant has colic.
   b. The infant's length and weight are above the 85th percentile.
   c. The infant has a severe diaper rash.
   d. A port-wine stain is present on the infant's left thigh.

9. As the examiner palpates an enlarged lymph node, the patient complains of pain. This is an indication of
   a. an inflammatory process.
   b. Hodgkin disease.
   c. immature lymph node development.
   d. malignancy.

10. Which examination method is used to differentiate an enlarged lymph node from a cyst?
    a. Palpation
    b. Auscultation
    c. Biopsy
    d. Transillumination

11. Which of the following methods best describes how to assess supraclavicular lymph nodes?
    a. Place the patient in a supine position and ask the patient to hold his or her breath.
    b. Place the patient in the Trendelenburg position and then illuminate the lymph nodes with a bright light.
    c. Palpate deeply behind the clavicles as the patient takes a deep breath.
    d. Palpate lightly below the clavicles with the patient in a sitting position leaning forward.

12. The examiner notes enlarged tonsils in a young child. The examiner should recognize that this
    a. is an indication of a retropharyngeal abscess.
    b. may be an early indication of Epstein-Barr virus.
    c. is an indication that the child has lymphoma.
    d. may be a normal finding.

13. In addition to the head, neck, axillae, and inguinal area, the examiner may also assess lymph nodes in which location?
    a. On the palmar aspect of the hands
    b. In the popliteal region
    c. In the patellar region
    d. On the dorsum of the foot

14. A patient with tuberculosis is most likely to have which finding?
    a. Hard and fixed nodes
    b. Pulsating lymph nodes
    c. "Cold" lymph nodes
    d. Lymph node cysts

15. Which of the following is an assessment technique that can differentiate mumps from cervical adenitis?
    a. Palpating the angle of the jaw
    b. Palpating enlarged lymph nodes
    c. Noting painful lymph nodes
    d. Noting swelling of the face

16. What is the importance of assessing the lymph system and drainage pattern of the lymph system?
    a. The lymph drainage pattern tracks the disease course.
    b. It determines the rationale for the disease progress.
    c. Enlargement of a node may be a sign of pathology that is from a distance.
    d. The drainage pattern assists in identifying the type of pathology.

17. Mrs. Alberts presents to the office with a complaint of a swelling in her neck. What would you expect to feel if the lymph node was cancerous?
   a. Less than 0.5 cm in size and soft
   b. Nonpalpable lymph node
   c. Matted, firm, almost rubbery lymph node
   d. Lymph node matches the other side of the neck lymph nodes

18. Normal cervical lymph nodes are
   a. matted.
   b. tender to palpation.
   c. rubbery.
   d. smaller than 1 cm.

LEARNING OBJECTIVES

After studying Chapter 10 in the textbook and completing this section of the laboratory manual, students should be able to:
1. Conduct a history related to the head and neck.
2. Discuss examination techniques for the head and neck.
3. Identify normal age and condition variations related to the head and neck.
4. Recognize findings that deviate from expected findings.
5. Relate symptoms or clinical findings to common pathologic conditions.

TEXTBOOK REVIEW

Chapter 10: Head and Neck (pp. 184–203)

CHAPTER OVERVIEW

This chapter describes how to perform a health history and physical examination related to the structures of the head and neck. The anatomy and physiology of the head and neck structure are reviewed. Techniques to complete physical examination of the head and neck structure are examined, and special populations are discussed.

TERMINOLOGY REVIEW

Branchial cleft cyst—a congenital lesion formed by incomplete involution of the branchial cleft; the epithelial-lined cyst is usually solitary, painless, and located in the lateral neck; discharge may occur if associated with the sinus tract.

Bruit—a soft rushing sound that may be detected in the hypervascular thyroid.

Bulging fontanel—a condition of the fontanel that may indicate increased intra.cranial pressure from a space-occupying mass or meningitis.

Craniosynostosis—a condition that results from the premature closing of sutures before brain growth is complete; leads to a misshapen skull that is not accompanied by mental retardation.

Chloasma—facial discoloration common during pregnancy; also called the mask of pregnancy; this fades after delivery.

Encephalocele—a neural tube defect with protrusions of brain and membranes that cover it through openings in the skull; genetic component in families with history of spina bifida or anencephaly.

Exophthalmos— increased prominence of the eyes.

Facies—general appearance of the space and features of the head and neck, that when considered together, are characteristics of a clinical condition or syndrome.

Graves disease—an autoimmune condition in which antibodies to thyroid-stimulating hormone receptors lead to an overactive thyroid; includes a diffuse thyroid enlargement with prominent eyes (exophthalmos).

Hashimoto disease—autoimmune condition characterized by the production of antibodies against the thyroid gland, that often causes hypothyroidism.

Hyperthyroidism—overactivity of the thyroid.

Hypothyroidism—underactivity of the thyroid; more common than hyperthyroidism.

Macewen sign—percussion of the skull near the junction will be resonant; the sign associated with increased intracranial pressure after fontanels are closed.

Mastoid fontanel—a third (abnormal) fontanel located between the anterior and posterior fontanels; common in individuals with Down syndrome.

Microcephaly—a condition in which the circumference of the head is smaller than normal; associated with intellectual disability and failure of the brain to develop normally.

Molding—an abnormal shaping of the infant's head caused by the shifting and overlapping of bones during vaginal delivery.

Myxedema—skin and tissue disorder usually caused by severe prolonged hypothyroidism; characterized by coarse, thick skin; a thickening nose; swollen lips; puffiness around the eyes; slow speech; and weight gain.

Ossification—bone tissue formation; begins in sutures after brain growth is completed at about 6 years of age.

Salivary gland tumor—tumor in any of the salivary glands but most common in the parotid.

Sternocleidomastoid—the area extending from upper sternum to the mastoid process.

Thyroglossal duct cyst—a palpable cystic mass in the neck.

Thyroid—largest endocrine gland.

Tic—a spasmodic contraction of the face, head, or neck.

Torticollis—a condition in which the neck is twisted (also called "wry neck"); often the result of birth trauma or intrauterine malposition; acquired torticollis may be caused by tumor, trauma, palsy of cranial nerve IV, muscle spasm, infection, or drug ingestion.

Transillumination—procedure used to evaluate suspected intracranial lesion or increasing head circumference in infants.

Webbing—excessive posterior cervical skin, usually associated with chromosomal anomalies.

APPLICATION TO CLINICAL PRACTICE

Matching

Match each type of headache with its corresponding characteristic.

Type of Headache	Characteristic
_____ 1. Hypertensive headache	a. May be brought on by extreme anger
_____ 2. Classic migraine headache	b. May be brought on by alcohol consumption
_____ 3. Muscular tension headache	
_____ 4. Headache from temporal arteries	c. Associated with a well-defined prodromal event
_____ 5. Cluster headache	d. Begins in morning and decreases as day progresses
	e. Age of onset typically older adult

Anatomy Review

Identify the structures of the neck labeled on the illustration. Using the list of terms below the illustration, write the correct term in the blank next to the corresponding letter. Use each term once.

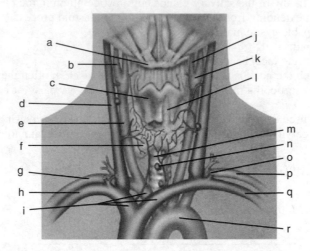

a. _____	External carotid artery
b. _____	Lymph node
c. _____	Carotid sinus
d. _____	Thyroid gland
e. _____	Hyoid bone
f. _____	Trachea
g. _____	External jugular vein
h. _____	Internal jugular vein
i. _____	Right subclavian artery
j. _____	Brachiocephalic artery and vein
k. _____	Internal carotid artery
l. _____	Common carotid artery
m. _____	Pyramidal lobe (thyroid gland)
n. _____	Arch of aorta
o. _____	Left subclavian vein
p. _____	Left subclavian artery
q. _____	Right subclavian vein
r. _____	Thyroid cartilage

Concepts Application

Complete the table below by listing the common characteristics of the physical appearance and demeanor of a patient with hyperthyroidism and a patient with hypothyroidism.

System or Structure	Hyperthyroidism	Hypothyroidism
Weight		
Emotional state		
Temperature preference		
Hair		
Skin		
Neck		
Gastrointestinal		
Eyes		

Case Study

Rob is a 44-year-old carpenter who comes to the emergency department complaining of a severe headache. Listed below are data collected by the examiner.

INTERVIEW DATA

When the examiner attempts to ask Rob about the headache, he cries out, "I can't take this anymore! It hurts too much!" His wife says that Rob has been getting these headaches a couple of times a day for the past week now—sometimes at night—so he has not been sleeping well. She also indicates that he had headaches like these about a year ago and that they lasted about a month. When the examiner asks Rob whether he experiences nausea or sensitivity to light, he replies, "No, I just get a stuffy nose." His wife says that Rob is constantly worried about whether—and when—the headache will come back because, as she says, "We don't know what is causing them, and nothing seems to help them go away." She says Rob feels like all he can do is hold his head and pray that the pain will stop.

EXAMINATION DATA

General survey: Alert, well-nourished man of average weight, in moderate distress. He is unable to lie still and paces the floor around the examination area, holding the left side of his head (over his eye and forehead).

Head and neck: Skull is intact, with no lumps, depressions, or tenderness. No abnormalities are found with facial structures. The head is centered on the neck; the trachea is midline. Thyroid is in midline position and of normal size.

1. What data deviate from normal findings, suggesting a need for further investigation?

2. What additional questions could be asked by the examiner to clarify symptoms?

3. What additional examination data should be assessed?

CRITICAL THINKING

1. What role does the technique of percussion play in the examination of the head and neck?

2. What role does the technique of auscultation play in the examination of the head and neck?

CONTENT REVIEW QUESTIONS

Multiple Choice
Circle the correct answer for each of the following questions.

1. In which group is a slight enlargement of the thyroid gland considered a normal finding?
   a. Infants
   b. Adolescents
   c. Pregnant women
   d. Native Americans or American Indians

2. Which of the following questions is most appropriate to ask a female patient with a suspected thyroid problem?
   a. "How much alcohol do you drink?"
   b. "Have you noticed a change in your sleep pattern or energy level?"
   c. "Do you have headaches?"
   d. "Are you currently menstruating?"

3. An infant with an alcoholic mother is admitted to the hospital with fetal alcohol syndrome. What assessment finding is consistent with this syndrome?
   a. Ear dysplasia
   b. Moon face
   c. Torticollis
   d. Thin upper lip

4. Which of the following findings in an older patient would be considered a normal process of aging?
   a. Narrowed palpebral fissures
   b. Pulsating fontanels
   c. Uneven movement of the tongue
   d. Fibrosis of the thyroid gland

5. Assessment of an infant's fontanels is best performed while the infant is
   a. calm and in an upright position.
   b. sleeping in a lateral position.
   c. supine and awake.
   d. held at a 45-degree angle.

6. A patient reports a severe headache accompanied by nausea, vomiting, and intolerance to light. These symptoms are consistent with which type of headache?
   a. Temporal
   b. Migraine
   c. Cluster
   d. Traumatic

7. A 6-month-old infant is brought to the clinic for immunizations. While examining the baby, the examiner notes that the anterior fontanel has not closed. What is the significance of this finding?
   a. This indicates a slight developmental delay.
   b. There may be a nutritional deficiency.
   c. This finding is consistent with hydrocephaly.
   d. This is a normal finding.

8. Preterm infants often have
   a. long, narrow heads.
   b. broad nose bridges.
   c. low-set ears.
   d. webbed necks.

9. The presence of a nodular thyroid is a normal finding in
    a. infants.
    b. adolescents.
    c. pregnant women.
    d. older adults.

10. Webbing, excessive posterior cervical skin, and a short neck are signs associated with
    a. Asian heritage.
    b. chromosomal anomalies.
    c. Cushing syndrome.
    d. malnutrition.

11. Transillumination of the skull should be performed
    a. in infants of mothers with diabetes.
    b. in infants with a history of traumatic birth.
    c. when an infant has a facial nerve palsy.
    d. in infants with suspected intracranial lesions.

12. Which of the following findings suggests an inflammation of the thyroid gland?
    a. Gritty sensation when the thyroid is palpated
    b. Movement of the thyroid when the patient swallows
    c. Vertical ridges palpated on the thyroid gland
    d. Swollen and red skin overlying the thyroid gland

13. A patient demonstrates asymmetry of the mouth. The examiner suspects a problem with the
    a. inferior facial nerve.
    b. thyroid gland.
    c. peripheral trigeminal nerve.
    d. salivary duct.

14. Mr. Andrews presents with complaints of a throbbing, unilateral pain in his head associated with nausea, vomiting, and photophobia characteristic of
    a. temporal arteritis.
    b. ophthalmic migraine.
    c. subarachnoid hemorrhage.
    d. migraine headache.

15. You are palpating a thyroid gland and note that it is enlarged bilaterally. What is your next step in the examination process?
    a. Listen for a bruit over the thyroid lobes.
    b. Examine the patient for enlarged lymph nodes.
    c. Check for a deviated trachea.
    d. Listen for a bruit over the carotids.

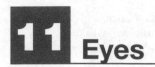 **Eyes**

LEARNING OBJECTIVES

After studying Chapter 11 in the textbook and completing this section of the laboratory manual, students should be able to:

1. Conduct a history related to the eyes and vision.
2. Discuss examination techniques for the eyes.
3. Identify normal age and condition variations related to the eyes.
4. Recognize findings that deviate from expected findings.
5. Relate symptoms or clinical findings to common pathologic conditions.

TEXTBOOK REVIEW

Chapter 11: Eyes (pp. 204–230)

CHAPTER OVERVIEW

This chapter focuses on the anatomy and physiology of the internal and external structures of the eye. Interviewing techniques to conduct a health history related to the eyes and vision are discussed as well as the impact for special populations. Physical examination techniques are examined, along with normal age- and condition-related variations found during eye examinations. Finally, this chapter evaluates symptoms and clinical findings related to common pathologic vision disturbances and eye disorders.

TERMINOLOGY REVIEW

Adie pupil (tonic pupil)—affected pupils dilated and reacts slowly or fails to react to light; responds to convergence, caused by impairment of post ganglionic parasympathetic apillaeons.

Amsler—a grid used to evaluate central vision.

Anisocoria—unequal pupillary size, more prominent in darkness, may be congenital.

Argyll Robertson pupil—bilateral, miotic, irregularly shaped pupils that fail to constrict with light but retain constriction with convergence.

Band keratopathy—deposition of calcium in the superficial cornea, most commonly in patients with chronic corneal disease; may occur in patients with hypercalcemia, hyperparathyroidism, sarcoidosis, syphilis, or renal failure.

Brushfield—white spots scattered in a linear pattern around the entire circumference of the iris, strongly suggest Down syndrome (trisomy 13).

Cataracts—opacity of the lens; most commonly resulting from denaturation of the lens protein caused by aging, which are generally central, peripheral cataracts that occur in hypoparathyroidism.

Confrontation—test for estimating peripheral vision, which is imprecise and can be considered significant only when it is abnormal.

Chorioretinal inflammation—an inflammatory process involving both the choroid and the retina; most commonly caused by laser therapy for diabetic retinopathy; this is also seen in histoplasmosis, cytomegalovirus, and congenital rubella infections.

Choroid—a pigmented, richly vascular layer that supplies oxygen to the outer layer of the retina.

Cornea—part of the eye that is optically clear, has a rich sensory innervation, and is avascular; it is part of the refractive power of the eye.

Corneal ulcer—a disruption of the corneal epithelium and stroma; associated with connective tissue disease, infection, and extreme dryness.

Cotton wool spot—ill-defined yellow areas caused by infarction of nerve layer of the retina.

Diabetic retinopathy (background)—a condition characterized by dot hemorrhages or microaneurysms and the presence of hard exudates as a result of lipid transudation and soft exudates as a result of infarction of the nerve layer.

Diabetic retinopathy (proliferative)—a condition characterized by development of new vessels as a result of anoxic stimulation; vessels grow out of the retina toward the vitreous humor; new vessels lack supporting structure of healthy vessels and are likely to hemorrhage.

Drusen bodies—appear as small, discrete spots that are more yellow than the retina.

Ectropion—the lower eyelid turned away from the eye; may result in excessive tearing.

Entropion—the eyelid turned inward, which results in corneal and conjunctival irritation with an increased risk of secondary infection.

Episcleritis—inflammation of the superficial layers of the sclera anterior to the insertion of the rectus muscles; occurs with an acute onset with mild to moderate pain and photophobia.

Exophthalmos—an increase in the volume in the orbital content, causing protrusion of the globes forward; most common cause is Graves disease; may be bilateral or unilateral.

Glaucoma—a disease of the optic nerve wherein the nerve cells die, producing a characteristic appearance of the optic nerve (increased cupping); visual field tests may show loss of peripheral vision.

Glaucomatous optic nerve cupping—physiologic disc margins are raised with a lowered central area.

Hemianopia—defective vision in half of the visual field; most common cause is interruption of the vascular supply to the optic nerve.

Hordeolum—an acute suppurative inflammation of the follicle of an eyelash that can cause an erythematous or yellow lump or sty caused by staphylococcal organisms.

Horner syndrome—interruption of sympathetic nerve supply to the eye, resulting in the triad of ipsilateral miosis, mild ptosis, and loss of hemifacial sweating; can be congenital, acquired, or hereditary (autosomal dominant).

Hypertelorism—eyes widely spaced apart; may be associated with craniofacial defects, including some with intellectual disability.

Iritis constrictive response—constriction of pupil accompanied by pain and a reddened eye, especially adjacent to the iris.

Lipemia retinalis—a creamy white appearance of retinal vessels that occurs when the serum triglyceride level exceeds 2000 mg/dL of the blood; seen in diabetic ketoacidosis and in some of the hyperlipidemic states.

Lens—a biconvex, transparent structure located immediately behind the iris; supported circumferentially by fibers arising from the ciliary body; highly elastic, and contraction or relaxation of the ciliary body changes the thickness.

Macula—also known as the fovea, it is the site of central vision; located approximately 2 disc diameters temporal to the optic disc.

Miosis—pupillary constriction, usually less than 2 mm in diameter.

Mydriasis—pupillary dilation, usually more than 6 mm in diameter.

Nystagmus—involuntary dysrhythmic movement of the eyes that can occur in a horizontal, vertical, rotary, or mixed pattern jerking nystagmus, characterized by faster movement in one direction, is defined by its rapid movement phase.

Papilledema—loss of definition of the optic disc; initially occurs superiorly and inferiorly and then nasally and temporally central vessels pushed forward.

Presbyopia—progressive weakening of accommodation, (focusing power); the major physiologic change that occurs after the age of 45 years; the lens becomes more rigid, and the ciliary muscle becomes weaker.

Pterygium—an abnormal growth of conjunctiva that extends over the cornea from the limbus; occurs more commonly on the nasal side but may arise temporally as well; more common in people heavily exposed to ultraviolet light.

Ptosis—drooping the upper eyelid; indicates a congenital or acquired weakness of the levator muscle or a paresis of a branch of the third cranial nerve.

Red reflex—a response caused by light illuminating the retina.

Retina—the sensory network of the eye that transforms light impulses into electrical impulses, which are transmitted through the optic nerve, optic tract, and optic radiation to the visual cortex in the brain.

Retinitis pigmentosa—an autosomal recessive disorder in which the genetic defects cause cell death (apoptosis) predominantly in the rod photoreceptors; earliest symptom is night blindness.

Retinoblastoma—an embryonic malignant tumor arising from the retina usually during the first 2 years of life; transmitted either by an autosomal dominant trait or by a chromosomal mutation gene on chromosome 13.

Retinopathy of prematurity—disruption of the normal progression of retinal vascular development in a preterm infant; results in abnormal proliferation of blood vessels called neovascularization.

Rosenbaum Pocket Vision screener—a handheld card used to test near visual acuity.

Sclera—a dense, avascular structure that appears anteriorly as the white of the eye; it physically supports the internal structure of the eyes.

Strabismus—a condition in which both eyes do not focus on the same object simultaneously, although either eye can focus independently; may be paralytic or nonparalytic.

Xanthelasma—a condition characterized by elevated plaque of cholesterol; commonly found on the nasal portion of the eyelid.

APPLICATION TO CLINICAL PRACTICE

Matching 1

Match each clinical finding with its corresponding associated factor.

Clinical Finding	Associated Factor
_____ 1. Adie pupil	a. Acute-angle glaucoma
_____ 2. Anisocoria	b. Congenital finding in 20% of normal population
_____ 3. Argyll Robertson pupil	c. Diabetic neuropathy or alcoholism
_____ 4. Mydriasis	d. Oculomotor nerve damage
_____ 5. Eye deviated laterally, downward	e. Neurosyphilis or midbrain lesion
_____ 6. Corneal arcus	f. Lipid deposition

Concepts Application 1

In the left column below, list the external eye structures in the order in which they should be examined. To the right of each structure, identify what specifically should be examined.

Structure	What Should Be Examined
1.	
2.	
3.	
4.	
5.	
6.	
7.	

Concepts Application 2

Referring to the following illustration, describe the position of the lesion based on disc diameter.

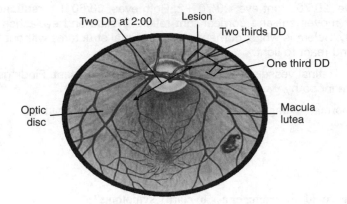

1. a. Location _____

   b. Length _____

   c. Width _____

Matching 2

Match each examination finding with its corresponding diagnosis.

Examination Finding	Diagnosis
_____ 1. Opacity in the lens	a. Lipemia retinalis
_____ 2. Dot hemorrhages or microaneurysms	b. Glaucoma
_____ 3. Eye vessels becoming progressively pink and then white as triglyceride levels rise	c. Cataract
	d. Background diabetic retinopathy
_____ 4. Characteristic appearance of the optic nerve—increased cupping	e. Retinoblastoma
_____ 5. Ill-defined mass arising from the retina in children	

Case Study

Andy is a 32-year-old single white male who has insulin-dependent diabetes mellitus. His reason for seeking care is a vision problem. Listed below are data collected during an interview and examination.

INTERVIEW DATA

Although Andy has been compliant with his treatment regimen, he has had poor control of his diabetes. He presents to the clinic with complaints of significant reduction in vision over the past couple of weeks. Andy tells the nurse, "I can't lose my vision because I won't be able to keep my job. If I can't see, I don't know how I will take care of my diabetes or how I will maintain my income."

General survey: Anxious, well-nourished male.

Eyes: Snellen test—left eye, 20/70; right eye, 20/70 +2; Both eyes, 20/60 +1; reduced peripheral vision. Normal extraocular movement and corneal light reflex. Eyelids and eyelashes symmetric. Conjunctiva clear bilaterally. Sclera is white; corneas clear. Lacrimal structures without tearing. Pupils are equal and round and react to light.

Internal eye examination: Retinal vessels hemorrhagic. New vessels present. Findings consistent with proliferative diabetic retinopathy.

1. What data deviate from normal findings, suggesting a need for further investigation?

2. What additional questions could the examiner ask to clarify symptoms?

3. What additional examination, if any, should the examiner complete?

4. What problem(s) does this patient have?

CRITICAL THINKING

1. A 5-year-old child is brought in for a routine physical examination. Describe what components of the eye examination are appropriate for a child of this age without specific eye or visual complaints.

2. While examining the eye, the examiner notes retinal vessels. How are arteries and veins differentiated?

CONTENT REVIEW QUESTIONS

Multiple Choice

Circle the correct answer for each of the following questions.

1. Which of the following is relevant information for a history and examination of a child's eyes and vision?
   a. Immunization history
   b. Growth milestones
   c. Birth weight
   d. Academic performance

2. Before instilling a mydriatic eyedrop, the examiner should
   a. assess the corneal reflex.
   b. observe the eye with focused light tangentially.
   c. assess intraocular pressure.
   d. observe the eye for vascular changes.

3. The examiner screens a 5-year-old child for nystagmus by
   a. assessing visual acuity.
   b. inspecting the macula of the eye with an ophthalmoscope.
   c. inspecting movement of the eyes to the six cardinal fields of gaze.
   d. palpating the globe while the child holds the eyelids closed.

4. Which of the following correctly describes the method to assess accommodation?
   a. Shine a light into the pupil; note constriction.
   b. Note constriction as gaze shifts from across the room to an object 6 inches away.
   c. Note ocular movement as the patient follows an object through the six cardinal fields.
   d. Cover one eye of the patient with a card; then remove the card, noting any deviation from a fixed gaze.

5. Which of the following should be used to test for near vision?
   a. Rosenbaum chart
   b. Snellen E chart
   c. Confrontation test
   d. Cover–uncover test

6. To visualize the macula, the examiner should ask the patient to
   a. blink the eye several times quickly.
   b. lie in a supine position.
   c. look directly into the light of the ophthalmoscope.
   d. direct his or her eye gaze on an object to the left and then to the right.

7. A 51-year-old patient tells the examiner, "My mother had glaucoma. What can I do to prevent myself from getting it?" Which of the following responses is most appropriate?
   a. "It is prevented by avoiding chronic eye irritation."
   b. "Limiting the exposure of ultraviolet light to the eye will prevent glaucoma."
   c. "Because it is inherited, you will eventually get it, and there is nothing you can do to stop that."
   d. "Although it can't be prevented, regular screening and testing assist in early detection."

8. Which of the following is considered a routine part of a newborn examination?
   a. Assessing red reflex
   b. Assessing extraocular movements with six fields of gaze
   c. Funduscopic examination
   d. Visual acuity

9. Which examination finding may be indicative of a retro-orbital tumor?
   a. Episcleritis
   b. Argyll Robertson pupil
   c. Unilateral exophthalmos
   d. Retinitis pigmentosa

10. A patient tells the examiner, "I have a loss of vision in the outer half of each eye." Which of the following underlying problems should the examiner consider?
    a. Diabetes
    b. Pituitary tumor
    c. Glaucoma
    d. Cytomegalovirus infection

11. Which of the following would be applicable to a family history?
    a. Eye dominance
    b. Pupil size
    c. Retinoblastoma
    d. Sty

12. Mrs. Carter has vision that, at best, is 20/210. Mrs. Carter is considered
    a. legally blind.
    b. mildly myopic.
    c. moderately hyperopic.
    d. unilaterally anisocoric.

13. Which of the following is the correct technique while performing an ophthalmoscopic examination? Examine the patient's right
    a. eye with your right eye and the left eye with your left eye.
    b. eye with your left eye and the left eye with your right eye.
    c. and left eyes with your dominant eye.
    d. and left eyes with your nondominant eye.

14. Failure to elicit a red reflex in a young child may indicate
    a. congenital glaucoma.
    b. myosis.
    c. retinopathy.
    d. retinoblastoma.

15. An examiner is most likely to observe pseudostrabismus in which of the following groups?
    a. Older adults
    b. Native American or American Indian infants
    c. Pregnant women
    d. Hispanics

16. A cobblestone appearance of the conjunctiva is most likely related to
    a. subconjunctival hemorrhage.
    b. allergic or infectious conjunctivitis.
    c. lagophthalmos.
    d. cytomegalovirus infection.

17. Mr. Barclay is a 48-year-old patient who presents to the office for follow up. On his eye examination, you note peripheral fundus changes and vessels that appear whitish. The most likely cause for these findings is
    a. floaters.
    b. lipemia retinalis.
    c. hypertension.
    d. glaucomatous optic nerve cupping.

18. Which of the following cranial nerves innervate the six muscles that control eye movement?
    a. II, III, IV
    b. III, IV, V
    c. III, IV, VI
    d. IV, V, VI

19. When you are examining the eyelid, you note ptosis on the right side. Which cranial nerve innervates the muscle that elevated the upper eyelid?
    a. CN II
    b. CN III
    c. CN IV
    d. CN VI

20. Mr. Kasey is a 57-year-old patient who presents to your office. During the eye examination, you note that his pupils are not equal in size; however, they react to light and accommodation. This is called
    a. anisocoria.
    b. Adie pupil.
    c. Hirschberg test.
    d. amblyopia.

12 Ears, Nose, and Throat

LEARNING OBJECTIVES

After studying Chapter 12 in the textbook and completing this section of the laboratory manual, students should be able to:
1. Conduct a history related to the ears, nose, and throat.
2. Discuss examination techniques for the ears, nose, and throat.
3. Identify normal age and condition variations related to the ears, nose, and throat.
4. Recognize findings that deviate from expected findings.
5. Relate symptoms or clinical findings to common pathologic conditions.

TEXTBOOK REVIEW

Chapter 12: Ears, Nose, and Throat (pp. 231–259)

CHAPTER OVERVIEW

This chapter begins with a review of the anatomy and physiology of the ears, nose, and throat, providing information regarding their integrity and function. The interviewing techniques used to conduct a health history related to the ears, nose, and throat are discussed. In addition, this chapter examines physical examination techniques related to the ears, nose, and throat. Age-specific variations of these techniques are also described. Clinical findings and symptoms of common pathologic conditions are examined, as well as age-related abnormalities.

TERMINOLOGY REVIEW

Acute otitis media without and with effusion—inflammation in the middle ear resulting in the collection of serous, mucoid, or purulent fluid (effusion) when the tympanic membrane is intact.

Acute pharyngitis—infection of tonsils or the posterior pharynx by microorganisms, often include group A beta-hemolytic streptococci, *Neisseria gonorrhoeae*, and *Mycoplasma pneumoniae*.

Cerumen—earwax, secreted by the apocrine glands in the distal third of the ear canal; provides an acidic pH environment that inhibits the growth of microorganisms; comes in two types—wet and dry—and it is a genetic trait.

Cheilitis—dry, cracked lips; may be caused by dehydration from wind chapping, dentures, braces, or excessive lip licking.

Cheilosis—deep fissures at the corners of the mouth; may indicate riboflavin deficiency or overclosure of the mouth.

Cholesteatoma—epithelial tissue behind the tympanic membrane that is often the result of untreated or chronic recurrent otitis media; as the epithelial tissue enlarges, it can perforate the tympanic membrane, erode the ossicles and temporal bone, and invade the inner ear structures.

Cleft lip and palate—common craniofacial congenital malformation; the result of the lip or palate failing to fuse during the embryonic development before the 12th week of gestation; the cleft may be unilateral or bilateral and may involve the lip, hard palate, soft palate, or all three.

Cochlea—coiled structure in the inner ear containing the organ of Corti; transmits sound impulses to the eighth cranial nerve.

Conductive hearing loss—hearing loss resulting from reduced transmission of sound to the middle ear; may result from an excess deposition of bone cells along the ossicle chain, causing fixation of the stapes in the oval window, cerumen impaction, or a sclerotic tympanic membrane.

Epistaxis—nosebleed.

Epstein pearls—small whitish-yellow masses at the juncture between the hard and soft palate.

Fordyce spots—bumps that may appear on the buccal mucosa and lips; ectopic sebaceous glands that appear as small, yellow-white raised lesions.

Frenulum—small fold of tissue that attaches at a midway point between the ventral surface of the tongue and the tip and attaches the tongue to the floor of the mouth.

65

Ménière disease—the triad of hearing loss, vertigo, and tinnitus; a disorder of progressive hearing loss; in some cases, it has a genetic mode of transmission.

Oropharynx—area of the throat that is located between the mouth and nasopharynx.

Ossicles—the three small bones of the inner ear known as the malleus, incus, and stapes that transmit sound from the tympanic membrane to the oval window to the inner ear.

Otitis externa—inflammation of the auditory canal and external surface of the tympanic membrane; also called "swimmer's ear"; produces intense pain on movement of the pinna and watery to purulent discharge.

Otitis media with effusion—inflammation of the middle ear resulting in the collection of serous, mucoid, or purulent fluid.

Otosclerosis—bone deposition immobilizing the stapes.

Peritonsillar abscess—deep infection in the space between the soft palate and tonsil; inflammation of Weber's glands resulting in cellulitis of the soft palate.

Pinna—projecting shell-like structure on the side of the head; the auricle.

Presbycusis—bilateral sensorineural hearing loss associated with aging resulting from changes in the inner ear or vestibular nerve.

Retropharyngeal abscess—life-threatening infection in the lateral pharyngeal space that has the potential to occlude the airway; most commonly occurs in children.

Rinne test—a hearing test that compares bone conduction with air conduction of sound.

Sensorineural hearing loss—hearing impairment that results from a disorder of the ear, damage to cranial nerve VIII, genetic disorders, systemic disease, or prolonged exposure to loud noise.

Sinusitis—bacterial infection of one or more of the paranasal sinuses.

Torus—bony protuberance on the midline of the hard palate.

Uvula—conical projection that hangs from the posterior margin of the soft palate.

Vertigo—the illusion of rotational movement experienced by a patient; often caused by a disorder of the inner ear.

Weber test—a screening test for hearing that tests the lateralization of sound.

Xerostomia—dry mouth.

APPLICATION TO CLINICAL PRACTICE

Matching

Match each clinical finding with its corresponding associated factors.

Clinical Finding	Associated Factors
_____ 1. Ménière disease	a. Dry mouth, systemic disease
_____ 2. Sinusitis	b. Fever, headache, nasal discharge, infection of one or more of the paranasal sinuses
_____ 3. Tonsillitis	
_____ 4. Xerostomia	c. Ear fullness, tinnitus; affects vestibular labyrinth
_____ 5. Presbycusis	d. Dysphagia, fever, fetid breath, referred pain to the ears
_____ 6. Otitis externa	e. Conductive hearing loss resulting from boney overgrowth of the stapes
_____ 7. Middle ear effusion	f. Epithelial growth that migrates through a perforation in the tympanic membrane
_____ 8. Cholesteatoma	g. Bilateral sensorineural hearing loss associated with aging
_____ 9. Otosclerosis	h. Inflammation of the middle ear resulting in a collection of serous mucoid or purulent fluid
	i. Infection of the auditory canal

Anatomy Review

Identify the structures of the middle ear labeled on the illustration below. Using the list of terms provided, write the correct term in the blank next to the corresponding letter. Use each term once.

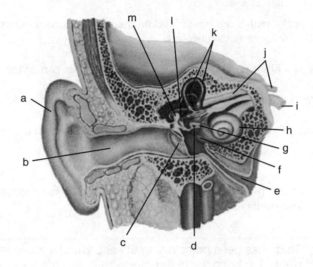

a. _____		Cochlea
b. _____		Malleus
c. _____		Cochlear and vestibular branch
d. _____		Round window
e. _____		Stapes and footplate
f. _____		Auricle
g. _____		Semicircular canals
h. _____		External auditory canal
i. _____		Eustachian tube
j. _____		Oval window
k. _____		Incus
l. _____		Facial nerve
m. _____		Tympanic membrane

Clinical Application

Fill in the blanks in the following statements, selecting the appropriate terms from the list below.

Darwin tubercle   Koplik spots
Epstein pearls   malocclusion

1. _____ are white specks with a red base found on the buccal mucosa opposite the first and second molars and may occur in a child with a fever or with rubeola.

2. A _____ appears as a blunt point projecting up from the upper part of the helix of the ear.

3. Improper position of the teeth is referred to as _____ .

4. On the roof of the mouth of an infant, _____ appear as small whitish masses and are considered a normal finding.

Case Study

Trudy is a 5-year-old Native American girl who was brought to the clinic by her mother. Listed below are data collected by the examiner during an interview and examination.

INTERVIEW DATA

The mother tells the examiner, "Trudy has been complaining of ear pain. She has been very hot and crying frequently." She adds, "I wanted to bring her to the clinic yesterday, but my grandmother told me I shouldn't." The mother continues, telling the examiner, "Trudy has been treated many times for this problem over the past several years by the medicine man. Last night I saw drainage from her ears. Grandmother told me this was a sign that the illness was being chased from the body. I did not know what it was, but I felt scared." The mother indicates that Trudy knows English but that the girl has never really talked very much.

EXAMINATION DATA

General survey: Small-for-age 5-year-old girl; quiet, flat affect. Does not look at the examiner; does not interact with the mother or the examiner.

External ear examination: Typical position of ears bilaterally. Left ear pinna red. Dried bloody drainage noted on left external ear and in left external canal. Cries when the left ear is touched. Right ear unremarkable.

Internal canal and tympanic membrane: Dried drainage noted in the left ear canal. Tympanic membrane perforated. Right ear tympanic membrane pearly gray; landmarks and light reflex present.

Hearing examination: Whisper test in right ear = correctly repeats four of five words; whisper test in left ear = none of five words repeated. Weber test = hears tuning fork in right ear.

1. What data deviate from normal findings, suggesting a need for further investigation?

2. What additional questions could the examiner ask to clarify symptoms?

3. What additional physical examination, if any, should the examiner complete?

4. What primary problems does the patient have?

CRITICAL THINKING

1. A mother brings her 6-month-old infant to the clinic and tells the examiner, "She has had a fever all night and has been crying for the past hour." The examiner looks in the baby's ears and notes that the tympanic membrane is red. How can the examiner differentiate redness caused by otitis media from redness caused by crying?

CONTENT REVIEW QUESTIONS

Multiple Choice
Circle the correct answer for each of the following questions.

1. When performing a Weber test, which of the following is considered a normal finding? The patient
   a. hears the tone equally in both ears.
   b. hears the tone better in one ear than in the other.
   c. hears sounds longer when conducted through air than when conducted through bone.
   d. is able to detect tones of varying frequencies and pitches from a tuning fork.

2. Which of the following best explains why infants and toddlers are at greater risk for ear infections than are older children and adults?
   a. Poorly developed immune system
   b. Immature tympanic membrane
   c. Wider, shorter, and horizontal eustachian tubes
   d. Excess deposition of bone cells along the ossicle

3. Which finding is most likely to suggest a foreign object in the nose of a young child?
   a. The mother states that the child plays with toys.
   b. The examiner notes a purulent discharge from the right side of the child's nose.
   c. The child has a foul-smelling odor from the nose.
   d. The child cries when lying down.

4. The examiner observes a blackish lesion on the top surface of the tongue of an adult patient. The patient indicates that his tongue is painful. Which question by the examiner would be helpful in explaining this finding?
   a. "Have you been taking antibiotics lately?"
   b. "Have you injured your tongue?"
   c. "Have you been diagnosed with mouth cancer before?"
   d. "When was the last time you brushed your teeth?"

5. Which of the following situations is an indication for transillumination?
   a. The patient complains of epistaxis.
   b. The patient has crepitus with jaw movement.
   c. The parotid gland is palpable and tender.
   d. The patient complains of pain over sinuses with palpation.

6. The examiner notes that a patient's tonsils are enlarged and that they touch the uvula. This is documented as
   a. 1+.
   b. 2+.
   c. 3+.
   d. 4+.

7. Which of the following statements made by a parent should raise the examiner's suspicion that the tympanic membrane of a young child has ruptured?
   a. "She has some bloody, yellowish-looking stuff coming out of her ear."
   b. "She has been crying all night but feels better this morning."
   c. "My child has had a fever and earache."
   d. "My child's earwax is dark brown."

8. Which of the following statements made by a 72-year-old patient would indicate a normal process of aging?
   a. "My tongue feels swollen."
   b. "My tonsils are large and sore."
   c. "Food does not taste the same as it used to."
   d. "I have white and black spots under my tongue."

9. Which of the following behaviors, as described by a parent, is most likely to indicate a hearing problem?
   a. "My 4-month-old baby does not seem to respond to loud noises."
   b. "My 5-month-old baby is babbling, but she is not yet saying any words."
   c. "Sometimes my 3-year-old does not pay attention to me."
   d. "When my 15-month-old baby is talking, I sometimes have a hard time understanding her."

10. An infant born weighing less than 1500 g is at risk for
    a. otosclerosis.
    b. hearing loss.
    c. cleft lip and palate.
    d. choanal atresia.

11. While examining the ear of a 6-week-old infant, the examiner observes a tympanic membrane lacking conical appearance and with a diffuse light reflex. These findings
    a. suggest a congenital abnormality.
    b. suggest a ruptured tympanic membrane.
    c. are classic findings for otitis media in a neonate.
    d. are normal.

12. Chronic sniffling, nasal congestion, nosebleeds, mucosal scabs, and septum perforation are signs of
    a. chronic allergies.
    b. cocaine abuse.
    c. fungal infection.
    d. turbinate hypertrophy.

13. Mrs. Williams presents to the office for a follow-up visit. On examination, you note deep fissures at the corners of her mouth and identify this as cheilosis. You know this is a result of
    a. xerostomia.
    b. riboflavin deficiency.
    c. Peutz-Jeghers syndrome.
    d. peritonsillar abscess.

14. Mr. Cruz presents for a physical examination. On examination, you note that the lower molars are distally positioned in relation to the upper molars. How would you classify this malocclusion?
    a. Overbite
    b. Class 1 malocclusion
    c. Class II malocclusion
    d. Class III malocclusion

15. The most important clinical signs for sinusitis in adults includes which of the following?
    a. Persistent cough, temporal headache, fever over 100°F
    b. Poor response to decongestants, postnasal drip, previous tonsillectomy
    c. Purulent nasal discharge, mandibular toothache, nasal allergies
    d. Maxillary toothache, purulent nasal drainage, poor response to decongestants

13 Chest and Lungs

LEARNING OBJECTIVES

After studying Chapter 13 in the textbook and completing this section of the laboratory manual, students should be able to:

1. Describe anatomy and physiology of the chest and lungs.
2. Organize interview questions pertinent to chest and lung examination.
3. Describe appropriate equipment used for chest and lung examination.
4. Relate inspection, palpation, percussion, and auscultation examination techniques to the chest and lungs.
5. Distinguish variations in the health history and physical examination among infants, adolescents, pregnant women, and older adults.
6. Analyze normal examination findings and relate to examination findings associated with various conditions of the chest and lungs.

TEXTBOOK REVIEW

Chapter 13: Chest and Lungs (pp. 260–293)

CHAPTER OVERVIEW

This chapter reviews the anatomy and physiology of the respiratory system for the purpose of keeping the body adequately supplied with oxygen. The health history and physical examination of the respiratory system are described. Age-specific variations in the chest and lung examinations are discussed in relation to normal findings in the adult population. In addition, examination findings are related to various conditions of the chest and lungs. Finally, this chapter evaluates history and physical examination findings for common abnormalities.

TERMINOLOGY REVIEW

Apnea—absence of spontaneous respiration; it may have its origin in the respiratory system or a variety of central nervous system and cardiac abnormalities.

Asthma (reactive airway disease)—small airway obstruction caused by inflammation and hyperreactive airways; acute episodes triggered by allergens, anxiety, cold air, and cigarette smoke.

Atelectasis—incomplete expansion of the lung at birth or collapse of the lung at any age; caused by compression from the outside or resorption of gas from the alveoli.

Biot respirations—irregular respirations varying in depth and interrupted by intervals of apnea but lacking repetitive pattern; associated with increased intracranial pressure, respiratory compromise, or brain damage at the level of the medulla.

Bronchiectasis—chronic dilation of the bronchi or bronchioles caused by repeated pulmonary infections or bronchial obstructions; frequently seen in cystic fibrosis.

Bronchitis—inflammation of the large airways; leads to increased mucous secretions; acute condition is usually caused by infection; chronic condition is caused by irritant exposure.

Bronchophony—greater clarity and increased loudness of spoken words.

Bronchovesicular breath sounds—typically moderate in pitch and intensity; heard over major bronchi.

Bronchiolitis—bronchiolar (small airway) inflammation leading to hyperinflation of the lungs; occurs most often in infants younger than 6 months old; usual cause is respiratory syncytial virus.

Cheyne-Stokes respiration—a regular periodic pattern of breathing, with intervals of apnea followed by a crescendo–decrescendo sequence of respirations; often associated with serious illnesses.

Chronic bronchitis—bronchial tube (large airway) inflammation that is usually a result of chronic irritation exposure; associated with a cough that may be productive.

Chronic obstructive pulmonary disease—nonspecific designation that includes a group of respiratory problems in which chronic cough and often excessive sputum production and dyspnea are prominent features.

Cough—a sudden spasmodic expiration forcing a sudden opening of the glottis.

Course crackles—loud, bubbly noise heard during inspiration not cleared by a cough.

Crackles—abnormal lung sounds, more often heard on inspiration; characterized by discrete discontinuous sounds; also called rales.

Croup—a syndrome that generally results from infection with a variety of viral agents, particularly the parainfluenza viruses; occurs most often in children between 1½ and 3 years of age.

Cystic fibrosis—autosomal recessive disorder of exocrine glands involving the lungs, pancreas, and sweat glands; thick mucus causes progressive clogging of the bronchi and bronchioles.

Diaphragmatic hernia—an abnormal opening in the diaphragm.

Egophony—increased intensity of spoken sound with accompanying nasal quality.

Emphysema—condition in which the lungs lose elasticity and the alveoli enlarge in a way that disrupts function; common in patients with the extensive smoking history.

Empyema—purulent exudative fluid collected in the pleural space.

Epiglottitis—acute life-threatening infection involving the epiglottis and surrounding tissues.

Fine crackles—high-pitched, discrete, discontinuous crackling sounds heard during the end of inspiration not cleared by a cough.

Hamman sign—mediastinal crunch; found with mediastinal emphysema; a variety of sounds include loud crackles, clicking, and gurgling sounds heard over the precordium; they are synchronous with the heartbeat and not particularly so with respirations.

Hemothorax—presence of blood in the pleural cavity.

Influenza—a viral infection of the lung; normally an upper respiratory infection caused by alterations in the epithelial barrier; an infected host is more susceptible to secondary bacterial infections.

Kussmaul breathing—deep and usually rapid respirations; the eponym applied to the respiratory effort associated with metabolic acidosis.

Medium crackles—lower, more moist sound heard during the middle stage of inspiration and not cleared by a cough.

Pectoriloquy—a whisper that can be clearly heard through the stethoscope; associated with consolidation of lungs.

Pleural effusion—presence of excessive nonpurulent fluid in the pleural space; sources of fluid vary and include infection, heart failure, renal insufficiency, connective tissue disease, neoplasm, and trauma.

Pleural friction rub—dry, rubbing, or grating sound, usually caused by inflammation.

Pleurisy—inflammatory process involving the visceral and parietal pleura; often the result of pulmonary infections or connective tissue diseases.

Pneumonia—inflammatory response of the bronchioles and alveoli to an infective agent, which can be bacterial, fungal, or viral; acute infection of the pulmonary parenchyma caused by different organisms.

Pneumothorax—presence of air or gas in the pleural cavity.

Pulmonary embolism—embolic occlusion of the pulmonary arteries; relatively common condition that is very difficult to diagnose; a major clue to pulmonary embolism is pleuritic chest pain with or without dyspnea.

Respiratory distress syndrome—a condition that develops in preterm infants as a result of surfactant deficiency.

Rhonchi—sonorous wheezes; loud, low, course sounds similar to a snore; most often heard continuously during inspiration or expiration.

Stridor—high-pitched, piercing sound heard during inspiration; it is the result of an obstruction high in the respiratory tree.

Tracheomalacia—a "floppiness" or lack of rigidity of the trachea or airway.

Tuberculosis—chronic infectious disease that most often begins in the lung but may have widespread manifestations.

Vesicular—low-pitched soft and short expirations heard over most lung fields.

Vocal resonance—sound of the spoken word as transmitted through the lung fields; usually muffled and indistinct in quality.

Wheeze—(sibilant wheeze) musical noise sounding similar to a squeak; most often heard continuously during inspiration or expiration; usually louder during expiration.

Auscultation Sounds

1. On the illustration below, label the locations of the lung sounds you would expect to hear with auscultation of the anterior chest using "B" for bronchial sounds, "BV" for bronchovesicular sounds, and "V" for vesicular sounds.
2. Mark the location of the manubrium with "M" and the angle of Louis with "AL."
3. Indicate the location of the costal angle with "CA."

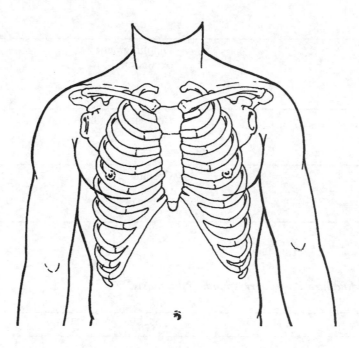

Examination Technique
For each clinical finding listed, identify the appropriate examination method that will elicit the finding.

Finding	Examination Method	Finding	Examination Method
Biot respiration		Bronchial	
Tactile fremitus		Rhonchi	
Cheyne-Stokes respiration		Barrel chest	
Dullness		Hyperresonance	
Vesicular		Wheezes	

Finding	Examination Method	Finding	Examination Method
Tympany		Tracheal tug	
Dyspnea		Crackles	
Bronchophony		Diaphragmatic excursion	
Vibration		Bronchovesicular	
Kussmaul breathing		Crepitus	

Matching

Match each examination finding with its corresponding diagnosis.

Examination Finding	Diagnosis
_____ 1. Airway reactivity triggered by allergens, anxiety, or upper respiratory infection	a. Bronchiectasis
_____ 2. Excessive nonpurulent fluid in the pleural space	b. Empyema
_____ 3. Inflammation of the mucous membranes of the bronchial tubes	c. Pulmonary embolism
_____ 4. Inflammatory process involving the visceral and parietal pleura	d. Asthma
_____ 5. Purulent exudate collected in the pleural spaces	e. Cystic fibrosis
_____ 6. Infection of the pulmonary parenchyma	f. Tuberculosis
_____ 7. Chronic infectious disease beginning in the lung with the tubercle bacillus	g. Pleurisy
_____ 8. Embolic occlusion of the pulmonary arteries	h. Bronchitis
_____ 9. Autosomal recessive disorder of the exocrine glands in children younger than 5 years of age	i. Pneumonia
_____ 10. Chronic dilation of the bronchi or bronchioles caused by repeated pulmonary infections	j. Pleural effusion

Case Study

Sharon is a 66-year-old woman presenting with symptoms of shortness of breath. Listed below are initial data collected during an interview and examination.

<u>INTERVIEW DATA</u>

Sharon says she has had breathing problems "for years," but now they are getting worse. She tells the examiner that she gets short of breath with activity, adding that she can do things around the house for only a few minutes before she has to sit down to rest and catch her breath. She says she can sleep only a couple of hours at a time. She sleeps best with two pillows at night, but on some nights, she just sits in a chair. Sharon does not currently use oxygen, but she thinks oxygen would help. She admits to smoking 1½ packs of cigarettes a day. She has never quit because she says she just can't do it.

<u>EXAMINATION DATA</u>

General survey: Alert and slightly anxious woman, sitting slightly forward, with moderately labored breathing. Skin is pale with slight cyanosis around the lips and in nail beds. Appears extremely thin.

Chest wall configuration: Chest is round shaped and symmetric with an increased anteroposterior diameter and costal angle greater than 90 degrees. Small muscle mass noted over chest; ribs protrude.

Breathing effort: Respiratory rate 24 breaths/min and labored.

Chest assessment: Chest wall expansion with respirations is reduced but symmetric. Chest wall tactile fremitus diminished. Rhonchi are auscultated throughout lung field. Lung sounds are diminished in lung bases bilaterally.

Vocal sound auscultation: Muffled tones auscultated.

1. What data deviate from normal findings, suggesting a need for further investigation?

2. What additional questions could be asked by the examiner to clarify symptoms?

3. What additional physical examination, if any, should the examiner complete?

4. What type of problems do you anticipate this patient will have?

CRITICAL THINKING

1. Louis Jackson is a 72-year-old man who is seen in the clinic for a routine examination. During the interview, Mr. Jackson tells the interviewer that he smokes. When questioned further, he indicates he has been smoking for "roughly 60 years." He states, "I started smoking cigarettes when I was about 14 years old. Until I was about 25, I smoked a pack maybe every 3 days or so. Then I started smoking about half a pack a day until the age of 40. Since that time, I've smoked almost a pack a day." Mr. Jackson adds, "I knew I should quit, but I never really wanted to very much. I decided that when I got up to a pack a day, I would never smoke more than that." Based on the information given, calculate Mr. Jackson's pack-year history.

2. Mr. Pena is a 41-year-old migrant worker from Mexico who comes in the clinic where you work. Through an interpreter, you learn that he has had a fever with night sweats, fatigue, frequent coughing with reddish sputum, and weight loss. What significance do these symptoms have?

3. Mrs. Marino tells you that all three of her children have had problems with coughing and some trouble breathing ever since they moved into a new apartment 2 months ago. She says they have not had fevers with these symptoms. What type of interview questions should be asked to further explore these symptoms?

CONTENT REVIEW QUESTIONS

Multiple Choice

Circle the correct answer for each of the following questions.

1. As the chest of a newborn is examined, bowel sounds are auscultated in the chest. Which of the following best describes the significance of this finding?
   a. A normal finding in newborns
   b. An abnormal but benign finding in children until 2 years of age
   c. Abnormal and possibly indicating an enlarged liver
   d. Abnormal and possibly indicating a diaphragmatic hernia

2. Which of the following patients demonstrates the highest risk factor for respiratory disability?
   a. A patient with a history of hypertension
   b. A child who has had a previous respiratory infection
   c. A patient with paraplegia
   d. An extremely thin female patient

3. An adult male patient complains of a "persistent cold that will not go away." He is a nonsmoker, and his skin color is normal. Which of the following is most important to this patient's history?
   a. Allergy tests and treatment plans
   b. Expectations for treatment and care
   c. Experiences with difficult breathing
   d. Previous sports injuries and rehabilitation

4. A health care professional is examining the chest of a 22-year-old woman who is 8 months pregnant. The patient has a wide thoracic cage. Which of the following best explains this finding?
   a. She may have lung disease, such as emphysema.
   b. She may be hypoxic and may require oxygen supplementation.
   c. She may be pregnant with twins, causing abdominal contents to be forced up and out.
   d. This is considered a normal finding with advanced pregnancy.

5. In which of the following conditions should the examiner expect the costal angle to be greater than 90 degrees?
   a. Chronic obstructive pulmonary disease
   b. Pneumothorax
   c. Infant respiratory distress syndrome
   d. Atelectasis

6. Which of the following findings indicates respiratory distress in a infant or young child?
   a. Respiratory rate of 30 breaths/min
   b. Irregular respiratory pattern
   c. Observation of sternal and supraclavicular retractions with breathing
   d. Auscultation of bronchovesicular sounds throughout the lung field

7. The examiner notes a diaphragmatic excursion of 4 cm on the right side and 8 cm on the left side. What do these findings mean?
   a. The patient may have pleural effusion.
   b. The patient may have a pneumothorax.
   c. Asymmetric findings are common in well-conditioned adults.
   d. This is a normal finding because the right lung is larger than the left lung.

8. During percussion, the patient holds his or her arms in front in order to
   a. expose maximum lung area.
   b. make the ribs protrude.
   c. prevent attacks of coughing.
   d. reduce discomfort.

9. Which of the following examination techniques is *not* typically done when examining the chest and lungs of a newborn?
   a. General survey
   b. Inspection
   c. Percussion
   d. Auscultation

10. The patient tells the examiner, "I have been coughing up a lot of yellowish green phlegm." The examiner should suspect
    a. viral infection.
    b. tuberculosis.
    c. pulmonary edema.
    d. bacterial pneumonia.

11. To best visualize subtle retractions on a patient, the examiner should
    a. place the patient in a supine position.
    b. stand directly behind the patient.
    c. ensure that the light source angles toward the patient.
    d. position the patient directly under a bright examination light.

12. Which of the following findings may indicate an intrathoracic infection?
    a. Malodorous breath
    b. Protrusion of the clavicle
    c. Clubbing of the nail beds
    d. Kussmaul respirations

13. Which finding is considered unusual for a newborn?
    a. Sneezing
    b. Coughing
    c. Prominence of the xiphoid process
    d. Nose breathing

14. In an older adult, which finding can occur in the absence of disease as a result of age-related changes of the chest or lungs?
    a. Hyperresonance
    b. Productive cough
    c. Asymmetric expansion of the chest
    d. Pulmonary infiltrate

15. A newborn infant has a small chest-to-head size ratio. This finding is usually associated with
    a. maternal diabetes.
    b. cocaine use during pregnancy.
    c. intrauterine growth retardation.
    d. a normal variation of chest-to-head ratio.

16. Hamman sign can best be heard when the patient is
    a. in a supine position.
    b. lying on the left side.
    c. sitting completely upright.
    d. positioned with the head elevated 30 degrees.

17. In addition to severe respiratory distress, which of the following findings may be indicative of a pneumothorax with mediastinal shift?
    a. Hemoptysis
    b. Pleural friction fremitus
    c. Vesicular lung sounds over the peripheral lung field
    d. Tracheal deviation away from midline position

18. A mother tells the examiner that her 2-year-old child has a cough that "sounds just like a bark." Given this history, what other findings should the examiner anticipate during respiratory examination?
    a. Wheezing and coarse crackles bilaterally
    b. Labored breathing and inspiratory stridor
    c. Hyperresonance with percussion
    d. Productive, blood-tinged, or "rusty" sputum

19. A 4-year-old boy is brought to the emergency department. The examiner notes Kussmaul respirations of 50 per minute. The child has no fever and no cough; good air movement is noted in the lungs with no abnormal breath sounds auscultated. Which of the following questions would be most helpful for the examiner to ask the parents?
    a. "What is his normal respiratory rate?"
    b. "What would you like for me to do for him?"
    c. "Do you think he may have swallowed a toy?"
    d. "Where do you keep your medications at home?"

20. The examiner should expect the ratio of respiratory rate to heart rate to be approximately:
   a. 1 to 2.
   b. 1 to 4.
   c. 1 to 6.
   d. 1 to 8.

21. A patient with long-standing chronic obstructive pulmonary disease has come to the clinic complaining that his breathing has been getting more difficult over the past couple of weeks. Which of the following questions would best help the examiner understand the hypoxia this patient is experiencing?
   a. "Do you think oxygen will help you?"
   b. "In what way has your activity level been affected?"
   c. "Do you have a new or different cough?"
   d. "Have you been taking your medications?"

22. A patient has atelectasis. What finding would lead the examiner to suspect that an undiagnosed tumor in the middle lobe of the right lung has caused this problem?
   a. Low-pitched grating sound heard during inspiration and expiration
   b. Hyperresonance in the right middle lobe
   c. Diminished or absent breath sounds in the right middle lobe
   d. Coarse crackles auscultated throughout the lung field

23. Which examination finding is consistent with emphysema?
   a. Decreased tactile fremitus
   b. Dullness with chest percussion
   c. Trachea in midline position
   d. An ammonia-like odor to the patient's breath

24. The most important clinical signs for pleural effusion include which of the following?
   a. Bronchophony—yellow, frothy sputum
   b. Paroxysmal dyspnea, decreased breath sounds
   c. Shallow, rapid respirations
   d. Dullness to percussion, tactile fremitus

25. Which of the following is a normal finding in the assessment of an older adult?
   a. Loss of elastic recoil
   b. Decreased chest expansion
   c. Thickened chest wall
   d. Paroxysmal dyspnea

14 Heart

LEARNING OBJECTIVES

After studying Chapter 14 in the textbook and completing this section of the laboratory manual, students should be able to:
1. Describe anatomy and physiology of the heart.
2. Identify age and condition variations related to the heart.
3. Describe interview questions pertinent to the heart examination.
4. Discuss inspection, palpation, percussion, and auscultation techniques used for examination of the heart.
5. Describe age- and condition-specific variations in examination findings of the heart.
6. Identify examination findings associated with various conditions of the heart.

TEXTBOOK REVIEW

Chapter 14: Heart (pp. 294–331)

CHAPTER OVERVIEW

This chapter describes the anatomy and physiology of the heart, including the main heart functions to circulate blood through the body and lungs. Interviewing techniques used during the health history and heart examination are reviewed. Physical examination techniques, such as inspection, palpation, percussion, and auscultation, are described, including age- and diagnosis-related variations. Finally, this chapter identifies and discusses symptoms and clinical findings associated with cardiac abnormalities.

TERMINOLOGY REVIEW

Acute rheumatic fever—a systemic connective tissue disease occurring after streptococcal pharyngitis or skin infection; the affected valve becomes stenotic and regurgitant.

Angina—chest pain described as a pressure or choking sensation substernal or into the neck; the pain, which can be intense, may radiate to the jaw or down the left or right arm.

Atherosclerotic heart disease—narrowing of the small blood vessels that supply blood and oxygen to the heart; caused by deposition of cholesterol, other lipids, and a complex inflammatory process.

Atria—small, thin-walled structures acting primarily as reservoirs for blood returning to the heart from the veins throughout the body.

Atrial septal defect (ASD)—a congenital defect in the septum dividing the left and right atria; a large ASD greater than 9 mm allows left to right shunting of blood.

Bacterial endocarditis—a bacterial infection of the endothelial layer of the heart and valves.

Cardiac tamponade—excessive accumulation of effused fluids or blood between the pericardium and the heart.

Congestive heart failure—a condition in which the heart fails to propel blood forward with its usual force, resulting in congestion in the pulmonary or systemic circulation; constrains cardiac relaxation, impairing blood return to the right heart.

Cor pulmonale—enlargement of the right ventricle secondary to chronic lung disease.

Diastole—the phase of the cardiac cycle during which the ventricles dilate, drawing blood into the ventricles as the atria contract and thereby moving blood from the atria to the ventricles.

Intrinsic—referring to the type of electrical conduction system that enables the heart to contract and coordinates the sequence of muscular contractions taking place during the cardiac cycle.

Mitral insufficiency or regurgitation—abnormal leaking of blood through the mitral valve from the left ventricle into the left atrium.

Myocardial infarction—ischemic myocardial necrosis caused by abrupt decrease in coronary blood flow to a segment of the myocardium.

Myocarditis—focal or diffuse inflammation of the myocardium.

Myocardium—middle layer of the heart; responsible for the pumping action of the heart.

Patent ductus arteriosus—failure of the ductus arteriosus to close after birth.

Pericarditis—inflammation of the pericardium; often the result of a viral infection.

Pericardium—tough double-walled, fibrous sac encasing and protecting the heart.

Point of maximal impulse (PMI)—the location where the apical pulse is most readily seen or felt.

Pulmonic valve—structure that separates the right ventricle from the pulmonary artery.

Purkinje fibers—fibers of the ventricular myocardium that are specialized cells for electrical conduction that conduct the electrical impulses in the heart.

Regurgitation—backward flow of blood.

Senile cardiac amyloidosis—a condition caused by deposits of amyloid, fibrillary protein produced by chronic inflammation or neoplastic disease deposition in the heart.

Septum—partition dividing the left and right heart chambers.

Sick sinus syndrome—an arrhythmia caused by a malfunction of the sinus node; occurs secondary to hypertension, arteriosclerotic heart disease, or rheumatic heart disease.

Sinoatrial node—a small mass of cardiac muscle fibers where the heart's impulse of stimulation originates.

Still murmur—an auscultatory sound occurring in healthy children 3 to 7 years of age; caused by the vigorous expulsion of blood from the left ventricle into the aorta.

Systole—the contraction phase of the cardiac cycle.

Tetralogy of Fallot—a syndrome consisting of four cardiac defects: ventricular septal defect, pulmonary stenosis, dextroposition of the aorta, and right ventricular hypertrophy.

Thrill—a fine, palpable sensation.

Ventricular septal defect—an opening between the left and right ventricles of the heart; some blood from the left ventricle goes into the right ventricle, passes through the lungs, and reenters the left ventricle via the pulmonary veins and left atrium.

APPLICATION TO CLINICAL PRACTICE

Anatomy Review

Identify the structures of the heart labeled on the illustration below. Using the list of terms provided, write the correct term in the blank next to the corresponding letter. Use each term once.

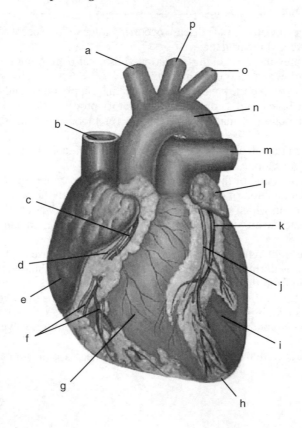

a. _____   Anterior cardiac veins

b. _____   Apex

c. _____   Arch of aorta

d. _____   Brachiocephalic artery

e. _____   Coronary sulcus

f. _____   Great cardiac vein

g. _____   Left atrium

h. _____   Left common carotid artery

i. _____   Left coronary artery

j. _____   Left pulmonary artery

k. _____   Left subclavian artery

l. _____   Left ventricle

m. _____   Right atrium

n. _____   Right coronary artery

o. _____   Right ventricle

p. _____   Superior vena cava

Concepts Application

Complete the following table by indicating where you would auscultate to locate each valve listed.

Valve	Where Would You Auscultate?
Tricuspid valve	
Mitral valve	
Aortic valve	
Pulmonic valve	

Matching

Match each examination finding with its corresponding diagnosis.

Examination Finding	Diagnosis
_____ 1. Increase in mass and lateral displacement of the left ventricle	a. Ventricular septal defect
	b. Angina
_____ 2. Bacterial infection of the endothelial layer of the heart	c. Congestive heart failure
_____ 3. Syndrome in which the heart fails to propel blood forward	d. Pericarditis
	e. Sick sinus syndrome
_____ 4. Inflammation of the pericardium	f. Aortic stenosis
_____ 5. Sinoatrial node dysfunction	g. Left ventricular hypertrophy
_____ 6. Elevated serum cholesterol	h. Acute rheumatic fever
_____ 7. Opening between the left and right ventricles	i. Bacterial endocarditis
_____ 8. Systemic connective tissue disease that commonly occurs after strepto- coccal infection	j. Hyperlipidemia
_____ 9. Substernal pain or intense pressure	
_____ 10. Thickening and calcification of the aortic valve	

Case Study

Howard Spivak is a 76-year-old man complaining of difficulty breathing. Listed below are initial data collected during an interview and examination.

INTERVIEW DATA

Mr. Spivak doesn't know exactly when his breathing difficulty started, but it has gotten noticeably worse the past couple of days. He volunteers at the church library three mornings a week and plays golf twice a week. However, Mr. Spivak says that this past week, he has "just felt too tired to do anything." He also says that he has not been able to sleep very well at night because of his breathing difficulty. He adds, "I keep coughing out this frothy-looking phlegm." Mr. Spivak denies taking any medications at this time. He says that he doesn't smoke or drink alcoholic beverages.

EXAMINATION DATA

General survey: Alert, cooperative, well-groomed man. Appears to be stated age. Breathing is mildly labored.

Vital signs: Temperature 98.8°F (37.1°C); pulse 120 beats/min; respirations 26 breaths/min; BP 142/112 right arm, 144/110 left arm.

Pulses: All pulses palpable 2+. No carotid bruits bilaterally.

Lower extremities: Skin warm and dry without cyanosis. Even hair distribution. 2+ pitting edema noted bilaterally. No lesions present.

82

Chapter **14** **Heart**

Neck: Jugular distention and pulsation noted with patient in supine position.

1. What data deviate from normal findings, suggesting a need for further investigation?

2. What additional questions could be asked by the examiner to clarify symptoms?

3. What additional physical examination, if any, should the examiner complete?

4. What type of problems do you anticipate this patient will have?

CRITICAL THINKING

1. Mrs. Martin tells you that her 2½-year-old son prefers to squat while watching TV rather than to sit on the couch or floor. What is the potential significance of this statement?

2. A 10-year-old girl is brought to the clinic by her mother. The mother tells the examiner that the girl has been very tired and short of breath and that she has been running a low-grade fever. These symptoms have been getting progressively worse over the past few weeks. The only significant health history is treatment for strep throat last month. What, specifically, should the examiner look for to aid in the diagnosis?

3. Mr. Yazzie is a 42-year-old Native American or American Indian with insulin-dependent diabetes mellitus (IDDM). He is seen in the clinic for a diabetic foot ulcer that does not heal. In what ways does IDDM increase Mr. Yazzie's risk for cardiovascular-related problems?

Multiple Choice

Circle the correct answer for each of the following questions.

1. Dextrocardia is a condition characterized by which of the following?
   a. The right side of the heart is enlarged.
   b. The heart is positioned to the right of the stomach.
   c. The heart is positioned to the right, either rotated or displaced.
   d. Blood glucose level in the heart is higher than in other organs.

2. While auscultating the heart of an obese patient, the examiner should expect the heart sounds to be
   a. louder and closer.
   b. softer and more distant.
   c. louder and more distant.
   d. softer and closer.

3. The examiner is unable to palpate a patient's apical pulse. In addition, the heart sounds are very faint to auscultation. What condition should be considered?
   a. Pleural or pericardial fluid
   b. Congestive heart failure
   c. Mitral valve regurgitation
   d. ASD

4. What disease process should the examiner consider if a patient reports a several-week history of fever and shows clinical symptoms of congestive heart failure?
   a. Bacterial endocarditis
   b. Infarction
   c. Myocarditis
   d. Cardiac tamponade

5. Which of the following occurs in the body to accommodate the increased maternal blood volume in a pregnant woman?
   a. The heart rate drops to deal with greater cardiac output.
   b. The plasma volume decreases to allow for more erythrocytes.
   c. The heart is shifted in position toward a more horizontal orientation.

6. The examiner suspects that a patient has pulmonary hypertension. What examination findings are consistent with this?
   a. Decreased intensity of S1 heart sounds; increased intensity of S2 heart sounds
   b. A thrill palpated in the area of apex
   c. Paradoxic splitting of S1 and S2 heart sounds
   d. Pericardial friction rub

7. Which of the following cardiac changes occurs at birth in the normal child?
   a. The foramen ovale opens.
   b. Pressure in the right atrium rises.
   c. The ductus arteriosus closes.
   d. The relative mass of the left ventricle decreases.

8. In most adults, the apical impulse should be visible at the
   a. midaxillary line in the fifth right intercostal space.
   b. sternal notch.
   c. midclavicular line in the fifth left intercostal space.
   d. costovertebral angle.

9. While palpating the precordium, a heave is identified, with lateral displacement of the apical pulse. Such a finding may indicate
   a. mitral regurgitation.
   b. aortic stenosis.
   c. left ventricular enlargement.
   d. pericarditis.

10. A thrill generally indicates which of the following?
    a. A disturbance in the electrical conductivity of the heart
    b. A disruption of blood flow related to a defect of closure in the semilunar valves
    c. The presence of significant infection of the myocardium
    d. Pulmonary hypotension

11. Because percussion has a limited value in determining heart size, left ventricular size is more accurately determined by
    a. auscultating the heart sounds.
    b. locating the apical pulse or PMI.
    c. palpating the left sternal border.
    d. palpating the heart base.

12. Which of the following may be easily mistaken for cardiac-generated sounds?
    a. Bowel sounds
    b. Pulmonary insufficiency
    c. Pericardial friction rub
    d. Tracheal shifting

13. Cardiac tamponade is
    a. sudden in onset and requires immediate intervention.
    b. easily detected by auscultation.
    c. the result of excessive accumulation of fluid between the pericardium and the myocardium.
    d. characterized by excessive cardiac relaxation, increased blood pressure, and bounding pulse.

14. In the presence of heart failure, which age group is most likely to exhibit liver enlargement before pulmonary edema?
    a. Infants
    b. Children
    c. Adolescents
    d. Older adults

15. During cardiac auscultation, the examiner notes a midsystolic murmur with a medium pitch; a coarse thrill is palpated as well. These findings are consistent with which condition?
    a. Aortic stenosis
    b. Aortic regurgitation
    c. Pulmonic stenosis
    d. Mitral stenosis

16. Which of the following reports made by a patient suggests compromised cardiac output?
    a. "My heart pounds hard after going upstairs, but it settles down after I rest a minute."
    b. "My right foot hurts a lot. I have also noticed it is colder and darker than the left foot."
    c. "I have been really tired lately. By evening, I am too tired to do anything but lie down."
    d. "I keep getting sores on my legs and feet that take forever to heal."

17. Which of the following cardiovascular findings would be considered normal for a woman who is 8 months' pregnant?
    a. The heart position shifts up and to the left; the apex moves laterally.
    b. Percussion reveals a decrease in left ventricular size.
    c. Assessment of the lower legs reveal 3+ pitting edema.
    d. Blood pressure is 150/118 mm Hg.

18. Which principle helps the examiner determine where heart sounds are best heard?
    a. The Doppler effect diminishes the sound over time.
    b. Sound is transmitted in the direction of blood flow.
    c. Accumulation of fluid magnifies the intensity of sound.
    d. Duration of sound varies directly with frequency.

19. S_2 is
    a. the result of opening of the atrioventricular valves.
    b. the beginning of systole.
    c. best heard in the mitral area.
    d. of higher pitch and shorter duration than S_1.

20. Splitting of heart sounds is
    a. an unexpected event that should be further evaluated.
    b. the result of opening of the valves during exhalation.
    c. greatest at the peak of inspiration.
    d. caused by synchronization of valve closure.

21. To distinguish a murmur from respiratory sounds in an infant, the examiner could correctly do which of the following?
    a. Time the sound with the carotid pulsation.
    b. Distract the child with a moving toy.
    c. Ask the child to hold his or her breath.
    d. Use the flat side of the stethoscope to auscultate the child's chest.

22. On a young child, the examiner notes a systolic ejection murmur that is loud, harsh, and high in pitch heard over the second intercostal space along the left sternal border. What problem should the examiner suspect?
    a. Mitral valve prolapse
    b. Mitral valve stenosis
    c. Coarctation of the aorta
    d. ASD

23. To hear low-pitched filling sounds of the heart, the examiner should place the patient in a
    a. supine position and listen with the bell of the stethoscope.
    b. sitting position and listen with the diaphragm of the stethoscope.
    c. sitting position and listen with the bell of the stethoscope.
    d. left lateral recumbent position and listen with the bell of the stethoscope.

24. The heart rates of children
    a. are less variable than those of adults.
    b. may increase significantly with each degree of temperature elevation.
    c. react slowly to stress of any sort.
    d. tend to increase with age.

25. Common cardiac findings among older adults include which of the following?
    a. Vagal tone maintains the heart rate in a narrow range.
    b. Cardiac response to demands is rapid and effective.
    c. Apical pulse is more difficult to locate.
    d. Ectopic beats are usual and they signal serious pathology.

15 Blood Vessels

LEARNING OBJECTIVES

After studying Chapter 15 in the textbook and completing this section of the laboratory manual, students should be able to:

1. Describe anatomy and physiology of the blood vessels.
2. Identify age and condition variations in the blood vessels.
3. Describe interview questions pertinent to an examination of the blood vessels.
4. Discuss inspection, palpation, percussion, and auscultation techniques for examination of the blood vessels.
5. Describe age- and condition-specific variations in examination findings of the blood vessels.
6. Identify examination findings associated with various conditions of the blood vessels.

TEXTBOOK REVIEW

Chapter 15: Blood Vessels (pp. 332–349)

CHAPTER OVERVIEW

This chapter begins with a discussion of the anatomy and physiology of the venous and arterial structures of the vascular system. Age- and condition-related variations are described. Effective interviewing techniques to gather data for the health history related to the blood vessels are identified. The chapter also reviews the techniques of inspection, palpation, percussion, and auscultation, specifically in regard to examination of the blood vessels. Finally, abnormal history and physical examination findings are discussed in relation to various pathologic conditions of the blood vessels.

TERMINOLOGY REVIEW

Arterial aneurysm—a localized dilation, generally defined as 1.5 times the diameter of the normal artery caused by the weakness in the arterial wall.

Arterial embolic disease—a condition in which emboli may be dispersed throughout the arterial system; may be precipitated by atrial fibrillation, leading to clot formation within the atrium; instability of the clot can result in the dispersal of emboli; emboli can also be caused by atherosclerotic plaques.

Arteriovenous fistula—a pathologic communication between an artery and a vein; may be congenital or acquired.

Bruit—murmur or unexpected sound usually low pitched, and relatively hard to hear.

Claudication—pain resulting from muscle ischemia, characterized by a dull ache with accompanying muscle fatigue and cramps.

Coarctation of the aorta—stenosis of the aorta seen most commonly in the descending aortic arch near the origin of the left subclavian artery and ligamentum arteriosum.

Homans sign—the complaint of calf pain is a positive sign indicating thrombosis in the lower extremity.

Hum—a venous phenomenon without pathologic significance that is common in children.

Hypertension—elevated blood pressure, one of the most common diseases in the world.

Kawasaki disease—acute small vessel vasculitic illness of uncertain cause affecting young males more often than females; the critical concern is cardiac involvement in which coronary artery aneurysms may develop; symptoms include strawberry tongue and edema of the hands and feet.

Peripheral arterial disease—stenosis of the blood supply to the extremities by atherosclerotic plaques; most common cause of peripheral atherosclerosis.

Pitting—a type of edema characterized by a dent or depression that does not rapidly refill and resume its original contour.

Preeclampsia—a syndrome specific to pregnancy; determined by hypertension that occurs after the 20th week of pregnancy and the presence of proteinuria.

Raynaud phenomenon—exaggerated spasms of the digital arterioles (occasionally in the nose and ears) usually in response to cold exposure.

Regurgitation—backflow of blood as a result of incompetent valves.

Temporal arteritis—inflammatory disease of the branches of the aortic arch, including the temporal arteries.

Thrombosis—clotting within a blood vessel that may cause infarction of tissues.

Tricuspid regurgitation—backflow of blood into the right atrium during systole.

Varicose veins—dilated and swollen veins with a diminished rate of blood flow and increased intravenous pressure, varicose veins result from the incompetence of the vessel wall or venous valves or an obstruction in the more proximal vein.

Venous thrombosis—a blood clot that forms within a vein; can occur suddenly or gradually and with varying severity of symptoms; can be the result of trauma or prolonged immobilization.

Venous ulcers—ulcers that result from chronic venous insufficiency in which lack of venous flow leads to lower extremity venous hypertension.

APPLICATION TO CLINICAL PRACTICE

Anatomy Review

Identify the arteries and pulse sites labeled on the diagram by writing the correct term in the blank next to the corresponding letter.

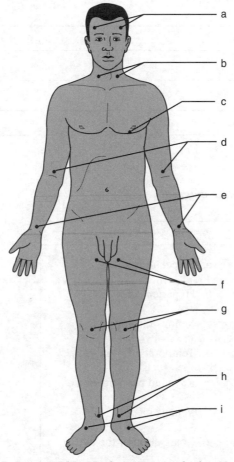

From Sorrentino SA, Remmert LN: *Mosby's Essentials for Nursing Assistants,* ed 5, Mosby, St. Louis, 2014.

a. _____	f. _____
b. _____	g. _____
c. _____	h. _____
d. _____	i. _____
e. _____	

Concepts Application Activity 1

Based on the location of pain, identify the probable obstructed artery.

Location of Pain	Probable Obstructed Artery
Calf muscles	
Thigh	
Buttock	

Concepts Application Activity 2

Complete the columns below by describing three characteristics that differentiate the pain of arterial insufficiency from the pain of venous insufficiency or musculoskeletal disorders.

Arterial Insufficiency	Venous Insufficiency or Musculoskeletal Disorders
1.	
2.	
3.	

Matching

Match each examination finding with its corresponding diagnosis.

Examination Finding	Diagnosis
_____ 1. Generalized inflammatory disease of the branches of the aortic arch	a. Preeclampsia
	b. Hypertension
_____ 2. Idiopathic, intermittent spasm of the arterioles in the digits	c. Venous thrombosis
_____ 3. Consistently elevated blood pressure (higher than 140/90 mm Hg)	d. Temporal arteritis
	e. Raynaud phenomenon
_____ 4. Tenderness along the iliac vessels and femoral canal	f. Venous ulcers
_____ 5. Holosystolic murmur in the tricuspid valve	g. Coarctation of the aorta
_____ 6. Congenital stenosis in the descending aortic arch in children	h. Tricuspid regurgitation
_____ 7. Hypertension that occurs after the 20th week of pregnancy along with the presence of proteinuria	
_____ 8. Chronic venous insufficiency in which lack of venous flow leads to lower extremity venous hypertension	

Case Study

Felice is a 32-year-old woman who presents with symptoms of pain in her fingers, with more discomfort in her dominant right hand. Listed below are initial data collected during an interview and examination.

INTERVIEW DATA

Felice began to notice changes in her hands about 3 months ago when she started a new job where she spends several hours a day at a computer keyboard. Since then, the pain has steadily increased, and she is alarmed about the development of a dark spot on the tip of the fifth finger of her right hand. Felice attends aerobic classes weekly but is not able to keep up with the class because of shortness of breath. She has smoked a pack of cigarettes daily for the past 10 years. Felice has a moderate alcohol intake of two to three glasses of wine per week. She is taking no medications at this time.

EXAMINATION DATA

General survey: Alert, cooperative, well-groomed woman who appears to be her stated age. Shortness of breath noted upon reaching the examination room but abated after 1 minute of rest.

Vital signs: Temperature 98.8°F (37.1°C). Pulse 100 beats/min on arrival to room; 76 beats/min after 5 minutes. BP 126/82 in both arms.

Pulses: All pulses palpable, 2+. Fingers on both hands cool to touch.

Lower extremities: Skin warm and dry; free of cyanosis or erythema. Hair distribution is even. No edema noted. No lesions present.

Upper extremities: Fingers cool, capillary refill sluggish. Dark lesion noted on tip of right fifth finger, 4 mm in diameter. Some reduced range of motion noted in both hands. Skin over the hands appears tight and probably contributes to the reduced range of motion.

Neck: Supple. No neck vein distention noted.

1. What data deviate from normal findings, suggesting a need for further investigation?

2. What additional questions could the examiner ask to clarify symptoms?

3. What additional physical examination, if any, should the examiner complete?

4. What type of problems do you anticipate this patient will have?

CRITICAL THINKING

1. Mr. Simmons reports that he has increasing pain in the calf of his left leg, which he began to notice after a long air-plane ride 1 month ago. He is 56 years old and has smoked a half a pack of cigarettes a day for the past 20 years. Examination reveals some redness and tenderness over the affected area. What do Mr. Simmons' symptoms suggest, and what is he at risk for?

2. Mrs. Porter comes to her routine prenatal check at 32 weeks' gestation complaining of difficulty with dizziness when she gets up from bed or from a seated position. What is the most likely cause of her symptoms?

CONTENT REVIEW QUESTIONS

Multiple Choice

Circle the correct answer for each of the following questions.

1. The carotid artery is considered the most suitable artery for evaluation of cardiac function because it
   a. is the largest artery in the peripheral vascular system.
   b. is the most pliable artery in the peripheral vascular system.
   c. is the most accessible artery close to the heart.
   d. has the thickest layer of smooth muscle within the vessel walls.

2. The purpose of the great vessels is to
   a. provide a reservoir for blood volume to be used in times of stress.
   b. circulate the blood to and from the body and the lungs.
   c. quickly and efficiently move blood in and out of the heart.
   d. send blood to the lungs for large-scale reoxygenation.

3. Pregnant women may experience palmar erythema and spider telangiectasis as a result of
   a. peripheral vasodilation with decreased vascular resistance.
   b. peripheral vasoconstriction.
   c. increased peripheral resistance.
   d. peripheral vascular resistance with diminished cardiac output.

4. The examiner suspects a patient has deep vein thrombosis. The examiner dorsiflexes the patient's foot, to which the patient reports calf pain. This finding is referred to as a positive
   a. Allis sign.
   b. Chadwick sign.
   c. Homans sign.
   d. Kehr sign.

5. Atherosclerosis, anemia, anxiety, and exercise are associated most with which type of arterial pulse?
   a. Alternating pulse
   b. Bounding pulse
   c. Labile pulse
   d. Paradoxic pulse

6. Which word best describes a 3+ amplitude pulse?
   a. Diminished
   b. Normal
   c. Full
   d. Bounding

7. Claudication
   a. is tissue necrosis caused by venous insufficiency.
   b. is pain that results from muscle ischemia.
   c. is characterized by sharp, tingling pain.
   d. occurs after exercise and during sleep.

8. Korotkoff sounds
   a. are best heard with the diaphragm of the stethoscope.
   b. begin with the end of diastole and end at the beginning of systole.
   c. are produced by turbulence of blood flow in an artery.
   d. occur within the auscultatory gap.

9. To determine pulse pressure, the examiner would correctly do which of the following?
   a. Add the systolic and diastolic readings.
   b. Palpate the radial pulse while occluding circulation with the blood pressure cuff.
   c. Subtract the diastolic from the systolic readings.
   d. Apply manual pressure on the brachial artery while auscultating the Korotkoff sounds.

10. Reliable indicators of hypertension are
    a. numerous measurements taken over a period of time.
    b. any readings of blood pressure in which the systolic pressure exceeds 120 mm Hg.
    c. sitting, standing, and supine readings of blood pressure.
    d. findings of diastolic blood pressure in excess of 80 mm Hg.

11. Postural hypotension should be evaluated in which of the following patients?
    a. An older woman taking antihypertensive medication
    b. A pregnant woman with increased plasma volume
    c. All children younger than the age of 6 years
    d. A middle-age male complaining of sudden onset of chest pain

12. In determining the jugular venous pressure, the examiner would correctly do which of the following?
    a. Apply manual pressure on the carotid artery while the patient forcefully exhales.
    b. Examine neck veins while occluding the brachial artery with the blood pressure cuff.
    c. Use light to supply tangential illumination across the neck.
    d. Have the patient lean forward from the waist and take a deep breath.

13. Varicose veins are characterized by
    a. dilation and tortuosity when the extremities are dependent.
    b. increased rate of blood flow to the extremities.
    c. decreased intravenous pressure.
    d. edema resulting from obstruction to a distal vein.

14. A condition that results in progressive ischemia caused by insufficient perfusion is
    a. Raynaud phenomenon.
    b. peripheral atherosclerotic disease.
    c. venous thrombosis.
    d. arterial aneurysm.

15. In which group is a jugular venous hum an expected examination finding?
    a. Older adults
    b. Pregnant women
    c. Native Americans or American Indians
    d. Children

16. The patient tells the examiner, "My left leg has been hurting a lot lately, especially when I move my foot up and down. It also seems more swollen than the other leg." Based on these symptoms, the examiner should suspect
    a. hypertension.
    b. venous stenosis.
    c. venous thrombosis.
    d. arterial insufficiency.

17. The examiner notes a prominent jugular vein with significant pulsations. These findings are consistent with
    a. right-sided heart failure.
    b. hypertension.
    c. cardiac ischemia.
    d. left ventricular hypertrophy.

18. The most common cause of venous thrombosis in children is
    a. congenital venous incompetence.
    b. atherosclerosis of deep veins.
    c. arteriovenous malformation.
    d. placement of venous access devices.

19. Hypertension in children is most often the result of
    a. Addison disease.
    b. renal disease.
    c. stress and anxiety.
    d. side effects of prescription medications.

20. Which of the following distinguishes musculoskeletal pain from the pain of vascular insufficiency?
    a. Onset during activity
    b. Increases with intensity and duration of activity
    c. May occur several hours after activity
    d. Quickly relieved by rest

LEARNING OBJECTIVES

After studying Chapter 16 in the textbook and completing this section of the laboratory manual, students should be able to:
1. Conduct a history related to the breasts and axillae.
2. Discuss examination techniques for the breasts and axillae.
3. Identify normal age- and condition-related variations of the breasts and axillae.
4. Recognize findings that deviate from expected findings.
5. Relate symptoms or clinical findings to common pathologic conditions.

TEXTBOOK REVIEW

Chapter 16: Breasts and Axillae (pp. 350–369)

CHAPTER OVERVIEW

This chapter begins with a review of the anatomy and physiology of the breast and axillae region. Interviewing techniques related to the breast and axillae are described. Physical examination techniques for the breast and axillae are described, and various age- and population-specific findings are discussed. A major focus of the examination in adults is identification of breast masses, skin, and vascular changes that could indicate malignancy.

TERMINOLOGY REVIEW

Antibodies—important constituent of colostrum in addition to protein and minerals.

Areola—pigmented area surrounding the nipple that should be round or oval and bilaterally symmetrical or nearly so; the color ranges from pink to black.

Colostrum—clear or milky white fluid expressed from a breast before milk production; colostrum is produced and accumulates in the acinus cells (alveoli); it contains more protein and minerals then does mature milk.

Cooper ligaments—a layer of subcutaneous fibrous tissue that provides support for the breast; these are suspensory ligaments that extend from the connective tissue layer through the breast and attach to the underlying muscle fascia, providing further support.

Duct ectasia—benign condition of the subareolar ducts that produces nipple discharge; the subareolar ducts become dilated and blocked with desquamating secretory epithelium necrotic debris and chronic inflammatory cells.

Fat necrosis—benign breast lump that occurs as an inflammatory response to local injury; necrotic fat and cellular debris become fibrotic and may contract into a scar.

Fibroadenoma—a benign tumor composed of stromal and epithelial elements; related to a hyperplastic or proliferative process in a single terminal ductal unit.

Fibrocystic disease—a condition characterized by the benign fluid-filled cyst formation caused by ductal enlargement, usually bilateral and multiple.

Galactorrhea—lactation not associated with childbearing, usually from elevated levels of prolactin, resulting in milk production.

Gynecomastia—unexpected enlargement of breast tissue in men.

Intraductal papillomas—benign tumors of the subareolar ducts that produce nipple discharge; epithelial hyperplasia that produce a wartlike tumor in a lactiferous duct.

Involution—the interval, usually about 3 months, after termination of lactation when the breasts decrease in size.

Malignant breast tumor—ductal carcinoma arising from the epithelial lining of ducts; lobular carcinoma originates in the glandular tissue of the lobules.

Mammogram—a common radiologic procedure used for breast examination; the sensitivity is 77%, and the specificity is 95%.

Mastitis—inflammation and infection of the breast tissue, most commonly from *Staphylococcus aureus*, most common in lactating women.

Montgomery follicles—follicles that are tiny sebaceous glands and may appear in the areola.

Nipple—centrally located on the breast and surrounded by the areola; the lactiferous ducts open.

Paget disease—disease that is a surface manifestation of underlying ductal carcinoma; migration of malignant epithelial cells from the underlying intraductal carcinoma.

Papillomas—small tumors of the subareolar ducts that produce nipple discharge.

Peau d'orange appearance—appearance of this indicates the edema of the breast caused by blocking lymph drainage in advance of inflammatory breast cancer; the skin appears thickened with enlarged pores and accentuated skin markings.

Premature thelarche—breast enlargement in girls before the onset of puberty from an unknown cause.

Tail of Spence—area where most malignancies occur in breast tissue.

Tanner staging—staging for sexual maturity.

Virchow nodes—lymph nodes considered to be sentinel nodes for signaling lymphatic invasion of carcinoma from the abdomen or thorax.

APPLICATION TO CLINICAL PRACTICE

Matching

Match each clinical finding with its corresponding associated factor or cause.

Clinical Finding	Associated Factor or Cause
_____ 1. Galactorrhea	a. Malignant breast tumor
_____ 2. Mastitis	b. Ductal enlargement
_____ 3. Fibrocystic disease	c. Possible sign of breast malignancy
_____ 4. Dimpling in breast	d. Administration of phenothiazines
_____ 5. Nipple retraction	e. Clogged milk duct
_____ 6. 2- to 3-cm subareolar duct lesion	f. Blocked subareolar ducts
	g. Red, scaling, crusty patch
_____ 7. Paget disease	h. Intraductal papillomas
_____ 8. Mammary duct ectasia	

Concepts Application

On the illustrations below, draw the direction of palpation the examiner would use for the (a) back-and-forth technique, (b) concentric circles technique, and (c) wedge technique.

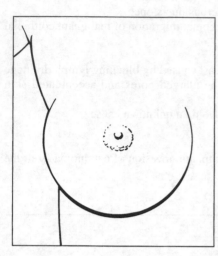 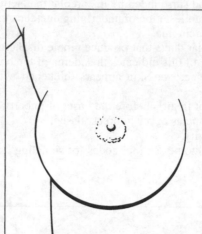 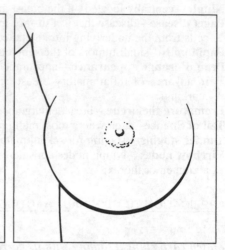

Case Study

Julie is a 46-year-old woman who comes to the clinic because she has discovered a lump in her left breast. Listed below are data collected during an interview and examination.

INTERVIEW DATA

Julie tells the examiner that she first noticed the lump about 9 months ago. Because the lump seemed small and did not hurt, she did not think it was much to worry about. Recently, Julie began noticing that the lump felt bigger and decided she better have someone look at it. Julie tells the examiner, "I just know it is not cancer because I am much too young and healthy. And if it is, I am not about to let some doctor mutilate me with a knife. I'd rather die than have my breast cut off." The examiner asks Julie whether she has noticed any redness or dimpling of the breast. Julie replies, "No, not really, but I don't pay attention to those sorts of things." She tells the examiner that she started having regular menstrual cycles at the age of 11 years and has not reached menopause. She has never been married and has no children.

EXAMINATION DATA

General survey: Very nervous, well-nourished woman. Is hesitant to expose her breast for examination.

Breast examination: Inspection reveals breasts of typical size with right and left breast symmetry. The skin of both breasts is smooth, with even pigmentation. The nipples protrude slightly with no drainage noted. The left nipple is slightly retracted. Significant dimpling is noted on the left breast in the upper outer quadrant when the arms are raised over her head. The right breast appears normal. Palpation of the left breast reveals a large, hard lump in the upper outer quadrant. No lumps or masses are noted in the right breast. The left nipple produces a clear, bloody-type discharge when squeezed; the right nipple is unremarkable.

1. What data deviate from normal findings, suggesting a need for further investigation?

2. What additional questions could the examiner ask to clarify symptoms?

3. What additional physical examination, if any, should the examiner complete?

4. What primary problems does the patient have?

CRITICAL THINKING

1. A 43-year-old female patient tells you her mother died of breast cancer and her 50-year-old sister currently has breast cancer. She is worried about developing breast cancer as well. Her gynecologic history includes menarche at age 11 years. She has one child, a 7-year-old son. She has no history of other pregnancies and no history of illness. List her current risk factors. Would you consider her to be at increased risk for breast cancer? Explain your rationale.

2. A 23-year-old woman requests information on how to perform breast self-examination. Describe the essential elements you would want to include in a teaching plan.

CONTENT REVIEW QUESTIONS

Multiple Choice

Circle the correct answer for each of the following questions.

1. A patient complains of a red rash on her breast. Which finding helps an examiner differentiate Paget disease from eczema? The lesion is
   a. unilateral.
   b. red.
   c. located on the nipple.
   d. raised and fluid filled.

2. Yvonne had a mastectomy of the right breast 2 years ago. Which of the following would assist the examiner with breast examination of this patient?
   a. Swelling, thickening, and small lumps around the mastectomy site are normal.
   b. The mastectomy site should be inspected but not palpated because of pain at the site.
   c. If malignancy recurs, it may be at the scar site.
   d. There is no need to examine the mastectomy site.

3. A woman in her third trimester of pregnancy asks the examiner about the drainage from her nipples. Her nipples are symmetric without redness. Which statement is true?
   a. Colostrum secretion is normal in the last trimester.
   b. Cultures should be taken to rule out an infection.
   c. Drainage from the nipple is an indication of a malignancy.
   d. The drainage is a sign of witch's milk.

4. While palpating the axilla, it is best to place the patient in a
   a. sitting position with the hands over the head.
   b. sitting position with the arms at the sides.
   c. supine position with the arms on the hips.
   d. lateral position with the arms at the sides.

5. A 58-year-old woman asks the examiner how often a mammogram is recommended for her. The best response by the examiner is:
   a. "Every 1 to 2 years if you have no symptoms."
   b. "Every 3 years."
   c. "Every 5 years if you have no symptoms."
   d. "Every 3 years if you have a family history of cancer."

6. A supernumerary nipple is found on a white newborn infant girl. Which of the following may accompany this finding?
   a. Increased risk for breast cancer as an adult
   b. Increased lactation volume as an adult
   c. Congenital renal or cardiac anomalies
   d. Mental retardation

7. A patient reports that she is concerned about the changes in her breasts that accompany her menstrual cycle. What should the examiner tell her about these changes?
   a. These changes are most likely to occur before and after the menstrual flow.
   b. These changes are alarming and might signal the development of a malignancy.
   c. These changes are a common response to hormonal changes during the menstrual cycle.
   d. Changes are most noticeable during the week after menstrual flow.

8. Which of the following is the correct position in which to place a patient for breast palpation?
   a. Supine with the arms at the sides and a pillow under the neck
   b. Supine with the arm over the head and a small pillow under the shoulder of the side being assessed
   c. Left lateral position with the arm bent backward
   d. Sitting slightly forward with the breasts hanging away from the chest; the hands on the hips

9. Which statement made by a 37-year-old woman would make the examiner suspect fibrocystic disease?
   a. "I have a lump in my breast that is not tender."
   b. "My right breast is larger than my left breast."
   c. "My nipples are darker than before my baby was born."
   d. "I feel a lump before my period."

10. A patient, 3 weeks postpartum, tells the examiner that she is currently breastfeeding but might stop because her nipples are sore. The examiner observes dry and cracked nipples. Which of the following questions would be helpful in gaining information relevant to treating the problem?
    a. "Do you pump your breasts?"
    b. "How do you clean your breasts?"
    c. "Have you been able to bond with your infant?"
    d. "What medications have you been taking?"

11. In an older man, gynecomastia may be secondary to
    a. a decrease in physical activity.
    b. increased lactiferous duct glands.
    c. lymphatic engorgement.
    d. a decrease in testosterone.

12. Symptoms consistent with underlying ductal malignancy include
    a. erythema, heat, and pain over and around one nipple.
    b. red, scaling, crusty patch on one nipple.
    c. bilateral inflammation; tenderness; and sticky, multicolored nipple discharge.
    d. gynecomastia and a deepening color of the nipple.

13. While examining the breast of a 52-year-old woman, the examiner notes nipple discharge. Which of the following diagnostic tests would be appropriate?
    a. Cytologic examination of the discharge
    b. Culture and sensitivity examination of the discharge
    c. White blood cell count
    d. Estrogen level

14. While performing a breast examination on a 68-year-old woman, the examiner would expect which of the following findings?
    a. The breast tissue has multiple large, firm lumps in it.
    b. The breast tissue has a granular feel to it.
    c. The tail of Spence is no longer observed.
    d. The axillary lymph nodes are enlarged.

15. Mrs. West is a 28-year-old patient who is pregnant. On examination of her breasts, you would expect to find:
    a. peau d' orange.
    b. smooth contours on palpation.
    c. flattened nipples.
    d. dilated subcutaneous veins.

16. Which of the following represents the first sign of puberty in girls?
    a. Thelarche
    b. Menarche
    c. Proliferation of lactiferous duct
    d. Areolar elevation

17. A benign tumor of the subareolar duct that produces nipple discharge is
    a. Paget disease.
    b. intraductal papilloma.
    c. duct ectasia.
    d. galactorrhea.

18. Mrs. Harris, a 38-year-old woman, is diagnosed with mastitis. What is the likely causative agent?
    a. Staphylococcus *aureus*
    b. *Streptococcus* aureus
    c. *Neisseria gonorrhoeae*
    d. *Escherichia coli*

17 Abdomen

LEARNING OBJECTIVES

After studying Chapter 17 in the textbook and completing this section of the laboratory manual, students should be able to:
1. Conduct a history related to the abdomen.
2. Discuss examination techniques for the abdomen.
3. Identify normal age- and condition-related variations of the abdomen.
4. Recognize findings that deviate from expected findings.
5. Relate symptoms or clinical findings to common pathologic conditions.

TEXTBOOK REVIEW

Chapter 17: Abdomen (pp. 370–415)

CHAPTER OVERVIEW

This chapter discusses the anatomy and physiology of the alimentary tract, gallbladder, pancreas, spleen, kidneys, ureters, and bladder. Specific variations related to age groups and special populations are reviewed. History and physical examination findings that deviate from normal findings are correlated to common pathologic conditions. During the abdominal examination, pay careful attention to the patient's comfort level and degree of distress.

TERMINOLOGY REVIEW

Acute glomerulonephritis—inflammation of the capillary loops of the renal glomeruli; results from immune complex deposition or formation.

Acute pancreatitis—an acute inflammatory process in which release of pancreatic enzymes results in glandular autodigestion; there are several known causes, including biliary disease and chronic alcohol use.

Acute renal failure—a sudden impairment of renal function over hours to days, resulting in an acute uremic episode; the most common clinical laboratory finding is a rise in the serum creatinine concentration.

Ascites—a pathologic increase in fluid in the peritoneal cavity; may be suspected in the patient with risk factors.

Ballottement—a palpation technique used to assess an organ or a mass.

Biliary atresia—a congenital obstruction or absence of some or all of the bile duct system, resulting in bile flow obstruction; most have complete absence of the entire extrahepatic biliary tree.

Borborygmi—loud, prolonged gurgles.

Cholecystitis—an inflammatory process of the gallbladder most commonly caused by obstruction of the cystic duct from cholelithiasis, which may be either acute or chronic.

Cholelithiasis—stone formation in the gallbladder that occurs when certain substances reach a high concentration in bile and produce crystals.

Chronic pancreatitis—a chronic inflammatory process of the pancreas characterized by irreversible morphologic changes resulting in atrophy, fibrosis, and pancreatic calcifications.

Cirrhosis—a diffuse hepatic process characterized by fibrosis and alteration of normal liver architecture into structurally abnormal nodules.

Colic—spasmodic pains in the abdomen.

Crohn disease—chronic inflammatory disorder that can affect any part of the gastrointestinal tract; produces ulceration, fibrosis, and malabsorption; the terminal ileum and colon are the most common sites.

Diarrhea—frequent liquid or loose stools lasting less than 4 weeks in duration; usually abrupt in onset and lasting less than 2 weeks.

Diverticular disease—a disease characterized by the presence of saclike mucosal outpouchings through colonic muscle; may involve any part of the gastrointestinal tract.

Duodenal ulcer—chronic circumscribed break in the duodenal mucosa that scars with healing; may develop from infection with Helicobacter pylori and increased gastric acid.

Fecal incontinence—inability to control bowel movements, leading to leakage of stool; associated with three major causes: fecal impaction, underlying disease, and neurogenic disorder.

Gastroesophageal reflux disease—backward flow of gastric contents, which are typically acidic, into the esophagus.

Hemolytic uremic syndrome—triad of microangiopathic hemolytic anemia, thrombocytopenia, and uremia; one of the most common causes of acute renal failure in children.

Hepatitis—inflammatory process of the liver characterized by diffuse or patchy hepatocellular necrosis, usually caused by viral infection, alcohol, drugs, or toxins.

Hiatal hernia with esophagitis—condition in which part of the stomach passes through the esophageal hiatus in the diaphragm and into the chest cavity; very common and occurs most often in women and older adults.

Hirschsprung disease (congenital aganglionic megacolon)—primary absence of parasympathetic ganglion cells in a segment of the colon, interrupting intestinal motility; abnormal intestinal innervation results in the absence of peristalsis, which leads to accumulation of stool proximal to the defect and intestinal obstruction.

Hydronephrosis—dilation of the renal pelvis and calyces caused by an obstruction of urine flow anywhere from the urethral meatus to the kidneys; increasing ureteral pressure results in changes in the glomerular filtration, tubular function, and renal blood flow.

Intussusception—prolapse or telescoping of one segment of intestine into another, causing intestinal obstruction; commonly occurs in infants between 3 and 12 months of age.

Irritable bowel syndrome—disorder of intestinal motility.

Lipase—an enzyme that acts on emulsified fats.

Meconium ileus—a distal intestinal obstruction caused by thick inspissated impacted meconium in the lower intestine of infants; pancreatic insufficiency or pancreatic anomalies are thought to be contributing factors.

Meckel diverticulum—outpouching of the ileum that varies in size from a small appendiceal process to a segment of bowel several inches long.

Mesentery—fan-shaped fold of peritoneum that anchors the small intestine to the abdominal wall.

Necrotizing enterocolitis—inflammatory disease of the gastrointestinal mucosa associated with prematurity and immaturity of the gastrointestinal tract; the most common gastrointestinal emergency in neonates.

Neuroblastoma—a common solid malignancy of embryonal origin in the peripheral sympathetic nervous system; the cause is unknown, but genetic and environmental factors are proposed etiologies.

Nonalcoholic fatty liver disease—a spectrum of hepatic disorders (not associated with excessive alcohol intake) ranging from steatosis to cirrhosis and hepatocellular carcinoma.

Pepsin—an enzyme that acts to digest proteins.

Peristalsis—muscular contractions that move the products of digestion through the alimentary canal.

Peritoneum—serous membrane lining the abdominal cavity.

Primary hepatocellular carcinoma—a malignant disease of the liver that frequently arises in the setting of cirrhosis, approximately 20 to 30 years after liver injury or disease onset.

Pyelonephritis—infection of the kidney and renal pelvis.

Pyloric stenosis—hypertrophy of the circular muscle of the pylorus, which leads to obstruction of the pyloric sphincter; The cause is unknown, but an association has been found with the use of a erythromycin.

Pylorus—distal section of the stomach.

Reflux—backflow caused by relaxation or incompetence of the lower esophagus.

Renal abscess—localized infection within the medulla or cortex of the kidney.

Renal calculi—stones formed in the pelvis of the kidney as a result of a physiochemical process; associated with obstruction and infections in the urinary tract.

Resonance—sound obtained on percussion of a body part that can vibrate freely.

Scaphoid abdomen—a concave contour of the abdomen; a sign that suggests diaphragmatic hernia in the newborn.

Striae—commonly known as "stretch marks."

Tympany—low-pitched, resonant, drumlike sound obtained by percussing the surface of a large, air-containing body space.

Volvulus—twisting of the intestine, resulting in an obstruction.

Wilms tumor (nephroblastoma)—most common intraabdominal tumor of childhood; usually occurs around 2 to 3 years of age; Wilms tumor gene *WT1* is located on chromosome 11 and regulates normal kidney development.

Anatomy Review

Identify the structures of the abdomen labeled on the illustration below by writing the correct term in the blank next to the corresponding letter. Use each term once.

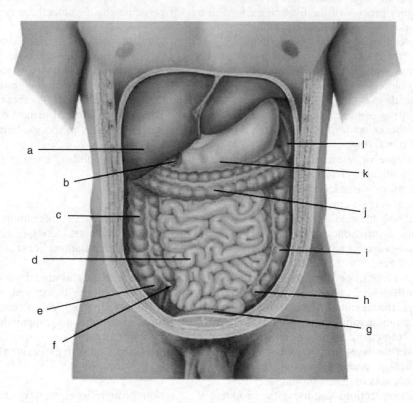

a. _____   Appendix

b. _____   Ascending colon

c. _____   Bladder

d. _____   Cecum

e. _____   Descending colon

f. _____   Gallbladder

g. _____   Liver

h. _____   Small intestine

i. _____   Sigmoid colon

j. _____   Spleen

k. _____   Stomach

l. _____   Transverse colon

Matching 1

Match each clinical finding with its corresponding abdominal condition.

Clinical Finding	Abdominal Condition
_____ 1. Knifelike pain	a. Intraabdominal infectious process
_____ 2. Dark yellow urine	b. Ulcer
_____ 3. Pain with gradual onset	c. Liver or biliary disease
_____ 4. Colic pain	d. Pancreatitis
_____ 5. Bruit	e. Renal stone
_____ 6. Burning pain	f. Aortic aneurysm

Concepts Application 1

Consider the two recognized divisions of the abdomen: four quadrants of the abdomen and nine regions of the abdomen (see p. 378 of the textbook). Referring to the illustration in the Anatomy Review exercise above, identify on the chart below the quadrant and the region where each of the listed abdominal structures are located. (Some structures are found in more than one quadrant or region.) The first one has been completed for you.

Structure	Quadrant	Region
Appendix	Right lower quadrant	Right inguinal
Colon		
Gallbladder		
Liver		
Pancreas		
Small intestine		
Spleen		
Stomach		

Concepts Application 2

Complete the table below to compare and contrast types of pain, abdominal signs, and associated symptoms or findings associated with the various conditions.

Condition	Type of Pain	Abdominal Signs	Associated Symptoms or Findings
Peritonitis	Sudden or gradual onset of generalized or localized pain described as dull to severe; increase in pain with deep inspirations		
		+Murphy sign	
Ectopic			Tender cervix, discharge, pregnancy dyspareunia, symptoms of pregnancy, spotting, hypogastric tenderness, mass on bimanual pelvic examination; with rupture: shock, rigid abdominal wall distention
	Sudden and dramatic LUQ, umbilical, or epigastric pain that may be referred to left shoulder		Fever, epigastric tenderness, vomiting
		+Kehr sign	Fever, hematuria

Concepts Application 3

Several sounds are heard on auscultation. For each sound listed below, identify the possible associated condition.

Sound of Auscultation	Possible Associated Condition
Increased bowel sounds	
High-pitched tinkling sounds	
Decreased bowel sounds	
Friction rub	
Venous hum	

Matching 2

Match each clinical finding with its corresponding diagnosis.

Clinical Finding	Diagnosis
_____ 1. Relaxation or incompetence of the lower esophageal sphincter	a. Cirrhosis
	b. Pyloric stenosis
_____ 2. Part of the stomach passing through the esophageal hiatus	c. Irritable bowel syndrome
_____ 3. Abdominal pain, bloating, constipation, and diarrhea	d. Cholelithiasis
	e. Gastroesophageal reflux
_____ 4. Ulceration, fibrosis, and malabsorption from an inflammatory disorder	f. Renal abscess
_____ 5. Left lower quadrant pain, anorexia, nausea, vomiting, possible constipation	g. Diverticulosis
	h. Hiatal hernia
_____ 6. Stone formation in the gallbladder	i. Crohn's disease
_____ 7. Destruction of the liver parenchyma	j. Acute renal failure
_____ 8. Impairment of renal function causing an acute uremic episode	
_____ 9. Localized infection in the kidney cortex	
_____10. Hypertrophy of the muscle of the pylorus	

Case Study

Katie is an 18-year-old young woman complaining of abdominal pain. Listed below are data collected by the examiner during an interview and examination.

INTERVIEW DATA

Katie tells the examiner the pain started yesterday evening and has gotten progressively worse. She describes the pain as "really bad." The pain is constant and located in her right lower abdomen toward her umbilicus. She says that her pain feels a little better if she stays curled up and does not move. She tells the examiner that she is in good health and that she has never had a problem with her stomach. Katie indicates that normally she has a good appetite and can eat anything. She says she ate breakfast and lunch yesterday, but by dinnertime she was nauseated and had no appetite. She has not eaten anything since. Katie denies any recent weight changes, but she says she would like to weigh about 5 pounds less than she currently does. She does not smoke or drink alcoholic beverages, and she takes no medication. Katie denies discomfort or problems with urination, describing her urine as "usual looking."

General survey: Alert and anxious young woman in moderate distress lying in a fetal position on the examination table with her eyes closed. Appears well nourished but not obese. Her skin is hot.

Abdominal inspection: Abdomen is flat and symmetric. No lesions or scars noted. No surface movements are seen except for breathing.

Abdominal auscultation: Bowel sounds absent.

Abdominal percussion: Tympany noted over most of abdominal surface; dullness over liver. Midclavicular liver span is 4 inches.

Light abdominal palpation: Demonstrates pain and guarding in right lower quadrant. Unable to palpate deep structures because of excessive abdominal discomfort. Demonstrates positive rebound tenderness in right lower quadrant.

1. What data deviate from normal findings, suggesting a need for further investigation?

2. What additional questions could the examiner ask to clarify symptoms?

3. What additional physical examination, if any, should the examiner complete?

4. What primary problems does the patient have?

CRITICAL THINKING

1. As you auscultate the abdomen, you should listen not only for bowel sounds but also for vascular sounds and a friction rub. List specifically what you are listening to and what abnormal findings may indicate.

2. Mr. Cane is a 46-year-old man with liver cirrhosis. You are preparing to check for ascites using a fluid wave technique. How is this particular procedure done, and what is a positive finding?

3. Cindy is a 24-year-old woman who is 7 months pregnant. Describe expected findings during an abdominal examination that are unique to pregnancy.

Multiple Choice

Circle the correct answer for each of the following questions.

1. Which statement suggests that a patient has a risk for contracting viral hepatitis A?
   a. "I am a health care worker."
   b. "I had a blood transfusion recently."
   c. "I have renal failure and have hemodialysis three times a week."
   d. "I have recently been overseas."

2. The examiner observes venous return on the abdomen of the patient that moves upward from the pubis to the chest. This finding should make the examiner consider
   a. portal hypertension.
   b. renal artery stenosis.
   c. inferior vena cava obstruction.
   d. mesentery arterial hypertension.

3. Which of the following questions would help an examiner determine whether a patient has an intraabdominal infection?
   a. "Where is the pain?"
   b. "Would you like something to eat?"
   c. "What does your urine look like?"
   d. "Is there a history of this problem in your family?"

4. Mrs. Cody is 36 weeks pregnant. She tells the examiner that her stomach muscle feels like it is splitting. A light protrusion of the abdomen midline is observed. This is recognized as
   a. abdominal dehiscence.
   b. swelling of the abdominal aorta.
   c. diastasis recti.
   d. umbilical herniation.

5. In which of the following patients would a slight pulsation in the epigastric area be considered a normal inspection finding?
   a. A very thin patient
   b. An obese patient
   c. A patient with ascites
   d. An older patient

6. The examiner palpates an organ in the left costal margin. Which technique should the examiner use to differentiate between an enlarged left kidney and an enlarged spleen?
   a. Auscultation, listening for renal bruit
   b. Auscultation, listening for abdominal friction rub
   c. Palpation, using indirect fist palpation to assess for tenderness
   d. Percussion, listening for dullness

7. A hiatal hernia is best described as
   a. a protrusion of abdominal contents through a weakening in the abdominal wall.
   b. a protrusion of the stomach through the esophageal hiatus of the diaphragm.
   c. an ulcer in the mucosa of the stomach that herniates into the peritoneal cavity.
   d. a herniation of the gallbladder into the cystic duct.

8. An examiner may wish to use a bimanual technique for abdominal palpation when
   a. palpating superficial organs.
   b. validating abdominal tenderness in the infant.
   c. meeting muscle resistance while performing deep palpation.
   d. determining the presence of excessive peritoneal fluid.

9. A history of chest pain is collected as part of an abdominal history because it may be
   a. associated with ulcers.
   b. caused by esophageal herniation and edema.
   c. perceived as esophagus and stomach pain.
   d. related to congenital abdominal defects.

10. You note that the midclavicular liver span of an adult male patient is 18 cm. With palpation, you note that the liver is enlarged, hard, and nontender. What do these findings suggest?
    a. Diverticulitis
    b. Ulcerative colitis
    c. Hepatitis
    d. Cirrhosis

11. The examiner is unable to palpate the liver or kidney on the patient. Which of the following techniques will help assess tenderness to these organs?
    a. Direct, continuous, firm pressure over the organ for several minutes
    b. Percussion for tympany
    c. Percussion for size
    d. Indirect fist percussion

12. In which age group is abdominal palpation easiest and most accurate?
    a. Young children
    b. Adolescents
    c. Young adults
    d. Older adults

13. Which of the following techniques is used to confirm the presence of abdominal ascites?
    a. Auscultation of fluid movement within the abdominal cavity
    b. Palpation of rebound tenderness
    c. Palpation of pitting edema on the abdomen
    d. Percussion of dullness over dependent areas of the abdomen

14. A 5-week-old male infant is brought to the clinic with a 2-day history of projectile vomiting. For what specific finding should the examiner assess?
    a. Abdominal pain with palpation
    b. Palpation of a small, round mass
    c. Auscultation of tinkering bowel sounds
    d. Auscultation of a bruit over renal artery

15. Which of the following examination findings is indicative of peritoneal irritation or appendicitis?
    a. Palpation of rebound tenderness
    b. Percussion of shifting dullness over the abdomen
    c. Auscultation of a bruit over the abdominal aorta
    d. Percussion of dullness over the suprapubic area

16. Which finding on a newborn infant suggests a congenital anomaly?
    a. The umbilical cord has one artery and one vein.
    b. The umbilical cord is thick.
    c. The umbilical cord is thin.
    d. There is a small mass around the umbilicus.

17. A 32-year-old female patient tells the examiner that when she goes running, she dribbles urine. Which type of problem should the examiner consider?
    a. Hydronephrosis
    b. Renal abscess
    c. Stress incontinence
    d. Overflow incontinence

18. A 61-year-old man has a presenting complaint of frequent constipation. He tells the examiner that there has been a change in his bowel movement habits—he gets constipated easily, the stool is very "skinny looking," and it is a different color than usual. He denies pain. What do these symptoms suggest?
    a. Diverticulitis
    b. Hepatitis B
    c. Colon or rectal cancer
    d. Pancreatitis

19. The functional ability of the gastrointestinal tract most severely affected by aging is
    a. motility.
    b. metabolism.
    c. digestion.
    d. catabolism.

20. Which rule states that the farther away from the navel abdominal pain occurs, the more likely it is to be of physical importance?
    a. Reglan rule
    b. Apley rule
    c. Applegate rule
    d. Romberg rule

21. An absence of bowel sounds in the right lower quadrant that indicates the possibility of intussusception is identified as which of the following signs?
    a. Grey Turner
    b. Aaron
    c. Dance
    d. Markle

22. Which of the following is the correct sequence for examining the abdomen?
    a. Inspection, auscultation, percussion, palpation
    b. Auscultation, inspection, percussion, palpation
    c. Inspection, auscultation, palpation, percussion
    d. Percussion, inspection, auscultation, palpation

23. Which of the following identifies Murphy's sign?
    a. Pain down the medial aspect of the thigh to knees
    b. Abrupt cessation of inspiration on palpation of the gallbladder
    c. Rebound tenderness and sharp pain when the right lower quadrant is palpated
    d. Right lower quadrant pain intensified by left lower clutching abdominal palpation

24. Peritoneal irritation is associated with which of the following signs?
    a. Aaron
    b. Balance
    c. Blumberg
    d. Dance

25. Abdominal pain radiating to the left shoulder may be indicative of which of the following?
    a. Appendicitis
    b. Intussusception
    c. Pancreatitis
    d. Splenic rupture

18 Female Genitalia

LEARNING OBJECTIVES

After studying Chapter 18 in the textbook and completing this section of the laboratory manual, students should be able to:

1. Conduct a history related to the female genitalia.
2. Discuss examination techniques for the female genitalia.
3. Identify normal age- and condition-related variations of the female genitalia.
4. Recognize findings that deviate from expected findings.
5. Relate symptoms or clinical findings to common pathologic conditions.

TEXTBOOK REVIEW

Chapter 18: Female Genitalia (pp. 416–465)

CHAPTER OVERVIEW

This chapter examines the anatomy and physiology of the internal and external female genitalia, including variations in adolescents, pregnant women, and older adults. Interviewing techniques for obtaining a health history related to the female genitalia and sexual history are described. In addition, physical examination techniques are described, as well as abnormal findings related to common pathologic conditions.

TERMINOLOGY REVIEW

Ambiguous genitalia—a newborn's genitalia are not clearly either male or female; usually caused by genetic abnormalities.

Atrophic vaginitis—inflammation of the vagina caused by the thinning and shrinking of tissues, as well as decreased lubrication; caused by a lack of estrogen during perimenopause and menopause.

Bartholin glands—glands located posteriorly on each side of the vaginal orifice, open onto the sides of the vestibule in the groove between the labia minora and the hymen.

Caruncle—a small, bright red growth protruding from the urethral meatus; most urethral caruncles do not cause symptoms.

Chadwick sign—a bluish discoloration of the cervix that normally occurs in pregnancy at 8 to 12 weeks gestation.

Clitoris—a small bud of erectile tissue, the homolog of the penis and primary center of sexual excitement, that is tucked between the frenulum and the prepuce.

Condyloma acuminatum—warty lesions caused by sexually transmitted infection with human papillomavirus (HPV); HPV invade the basal layer of the epidermis.

Cystocele—hernial protrusion of the urinary bladder into the vagina, sometimes exiting the introitus.

Endometriosis—the presence or growth of endometrial tissue outside the uterus; the pathogenesis is not definitive, but it is thought to be caused by retrograde reflux of menstrual tissue from the fallopian tubes during menstruation.

Genital herpes—a sexually transmitted infection of skin and mucosa most commonly caused by the herpes simplex virus type 2.

Hegar sign—softening of the cervix that is a sign of pregnancy, occurring at 6 to 8 weeks gestation.

Hydrocolpos—distention of the vagina resulting from an accumulation of fluid caused by congenital vaginal obstruction; obstruction usually caused by an imperforate hymen; or, less commonly, a transverse vaginal septum.

Hymen—a connective tissue membrane that may be circular, crescentic, or fibriated.

Infertility—the inability to conceive over a period of 1 year; contributing factors with women include abnormalities of the vagina, cervix, uterus, fallopian tubes, and ovaries.

Inflammation of Bartholin gland—a condition characterized by swelling of the Bartholin gland; commonly, but not always, caused by *Neisseria gonorrhea*.

Menarche—the onset of first menstruation, which usually occurs between 12 and 14 years of age.

Mittelschmerz—lower abdominal pain associated with ovulation; may be accompanied by tenderness on the side where ovulation took place that month.

Molluscum contagiosum—a viral infection of the skin and mucous membranes; considered a sexually transmitted infection in adults, in contrast to the nonsexually transmitted infection occurring in young children.

Myomas—common benign uterine tumors that arise from the overgrowth of smooth muscle and connective tissue in the uterus.

Ovarian cyst—fluid filled sac in an ovary; follicles undergo varying rates of maturation, and a cyst can occur as a result of hypothalamic–pituitary dysfunction.

Pelvic inflammatory disease (PID)—infection of the uterus, fallopian tubes, and other reproductive organs.

Premenstrual syndrome (PMS)—a collection of physical, psychological, and mood symptoms related to a woman's menstrual cycle.

Rectocele—hernial protrusion of part of the rectum into the vagina.

Rectouterine pouch—a deep recess formed by the peritoneum between the rectum and cervix (cul-de-sac of Douglas).

Salpingitis—inflammation or infection of the fallopian tubes, often associated with PID; can be acute or chronic.

Skene ducts—ducts that drain a group of urethral glands and open into the vestibule on each side of the urethra.

Syphilitic chancre—Skin lesion associated with primary syphilis; caused by the bacterium treponema pallidum.

Tubal pregnancy—ectopic pregnancy; pregnancy that occurs outside the uterus; most common site is the fallopian tubes.

Uterine bleeding—abnormality in menstrual bleeding and inappropriate uterine bleeding are common gynecologic problems.

Uterine prolapse—descent or herniation of the uterus into or beyond the vagina; the result of weakening of the supporting structures of the pubic floor.

Vaginitis—inflammation of the vagina.

Vulvovaginitis—inflammation of the vulvar and vaginal tissues; possible causes include sexual abuse or trichomonal, monilial, or gonococcal infection.

APPLICATION TO CLINICAL PRACTICE

Anatomy Review

Identify the structures of the female anatomy labeled on the illustration by writing the correct term in the blank next to the corresponding letter.

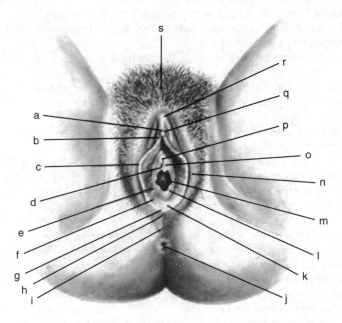

a. _____	Anterior commissure
b. _____	Anus
c. _____	Fossa navicularis
d. _____	Fourchette
e. _____	Frenulum of clitoris
f. _____	Glans of clitoris
g. _____	Greater vestibule of Bartholin duct opening
h. _____	Hymen
i. _____	Labium majus
j. _____	Labium minus
k. _____	Lesser vestibule of Skene duct opening
l. _____	Mons pubis
m. _____	Perineum
n. _____	Posterior commissure
o. _____	Prepuce of clitoris
p. _____	Urethral or urinary orifice
q. _____	Vaginal orifice
r. _____	Vestibule (identified twice)
s. _____	

Matching 1

Match each type of malignancy with its corresponding risk factors. Some risk factors apply to more than one malignancy.

Risk Factor	Malignancy
_____ 1. History of breast cancer	O: ovarian cancer
_____ 2. Smoking	C: cervical cancer
_____ 3. Infertility or nulliparity	E: endometrial cancer
_____ 4. High socioeconomic status	
_____ 5. Multiple pregnancies	
_____ 6. Average age, 46 years	
_____ 7. Multiple sex partners	
_____ 8. Early menarche	
_____ 9. Obesity	
_____ 10. Infection with HPV	

Matching 2

Match each diagnostic laboratory test with the type of instrument used to collect the specimen.

Diagnostic Test	Instrument Used
_____ 1. Gonococcal culture	a. Dacron swab
_____ 2. Endocervical cells	b. Wet mount with KOH
_____ 3. DNA probe for chlamydia and gonorrhea	c. Spatula
	d. Sterile cotton swab
_____ 4. *Trichomonas vaginalis*	e. Cytobrush
_____ 5. Both ectocervical and endocervical cells	f. Wet mount with NaCl
_____ 6. Candidiasis	g. Cervix brush
_____ 7. Ectocervical cells	

Concepts Application

Listed below are several alternatives to the traditional lithotomy position for pelvic examination. Compare these alternatives by describing each position and listing advantages or disadvantages of each.

Position	Description	Advantages or Disadvantages
Knee–chest		
Diamond shape		
Obstetric stirrups		
M-shape		
V-shape		

Case Study

Ms. Harris is a 33-year-old woman who presents to the urgent care center. Listed below are data collected by the examiner during the interview and examination.

INTERVIEW DATA

Ms. Harris tells the examiner, "I have a really bad pain in front of my butt. It hurts so much that I can't even wipe with a tissue after I go to the bathroom." She indicates that the pain started 2 days ago and is much worse now. When asked about her sexual activity, Ms. Harris says, "I have a guy that I'm with, but it's not exclusive or anything. We see other people and try not to be real serious."

EXAMINATION DATA

External: Typical hair distribution; urethral meatus intact; no redness or discharge. Perineum intact. Extreme pain response to palpation of vaginal opening. Swelling, redness, and mass detected on right side. Foul-smelling discharge noted.

Internal: Examination deferred because of extreme pain associated with inflammation.

1. What data deviate from normal findings, suggesting a need for further investigation?

2. What additional questions could the examiner ask to clarify symptoms?

3. What additional physical examination, if any, should the examiner complete?

4. What primary problems does the patient have?

CRITICAL THINKING

1. Lillian is a 42-year-old blind patient who requests a routine examination. How should the examiner approach this patient to best meet her needs?

2. Judy is a 16-year-old girl who is in the clinic for a school sports physical. How should her health history and an examination of her genitalia differ from that of an adult?

CONTENT REVIEW QUESTIONS

Multiple Choice

Circle the correct answer for each of the following questions.

1. Which finding is suggestive of PID?
   a. Enlargement of the ovaries
   b. Everted cervix
   c. Pain resulting from movement of the cervix
   d. Unilateral labial swelling, redness, and tenderness

2. Which finding would be of concern during an examination of an older female patient?
   a. Palpable ovaries
   b. Small and pale cervix
   c. Constriction of the vaginal introitus
   d. Absence of vaginal rugation

3. While palpating the introitus of the vagina, the patient jumps and complains of severe tenderness. A mass is palpated that is warm to touch. With which of the following problems are these clinical findings consistent?
   a. Cancer of the cervix
   b. Inflammation of the Bartholin glands
   c. A cystocele
   d. Acute genital wart infection

4. Which finding may be indicative of a pelvic mass? The cervix is
   a. pale in color.
   b. deviating to the right.
   c. protruding 2.5 cm into the vagina.
   d. pointing anteriorly.

5. The vagina, uterus, fallopian tubes, and ovaries are supported by four ligaments. Which of the following is a normal examination finding that evaluates this support?
   a. The uterus can be moved back and forth with manipulation.
   b. The patient is able to tolerate a wide-blade speculum during examination.
   c. The uterus and ovaries are easily assessed with bimanual palpation.
   d. The vagina and uterus are fixed and do not move with manipulation.

6. Which information is accurate and appropriate for an examiner to share with the patient following a Pap smear?
   a. "You may have heavier bleeding with your next menstrual period."
   b. "You may experience abdominal cramping for the next couple of days."
   c. "You will feel nauseated for the rest of the day."
   d. "You may experience mild bleeding or spotting over the next couple of hours."

7. A patient complains of pain; dysmenorrhea; and heavy, prolonged menstrual flow. Tender nodules are palpable along the uterosacral ligament. These symptoms and findings suggest
   a. PID.
   b. endometriosis.
   c. ectopic pregnancy.
   d. ovarian cancer.

8. An examiner plans to collect samples for cytologic studies during a vaginal examination. Before the examination, the examiner should lubricate the speculum with
   a. a water-soluble lubricant.
   b. topical anesthetizing ointment.
   c. warm water.
   d. vaginal secretions.

9. Symptoms associated with PMS are caused by
   a. ovulation.
   b. thickening of the uterine lining.
   c. elevations in body temperature.
   d. fluctuations in hormone levels.

10. When examining a woman who has had a hysterectomy, the examiner should
    a. delete the bimanual and palpation maneuvers.
    b. obtain a Pap smear from the suture line.
    c. omit cultures and specimens from the vagina.
    d. palpate internal areas before inserting the speculum.

11. A patient complains of urinary incontinence when she is active. Which associated finding might explain this problem?
    a. Hernial protrusion in the posterior wall of the vagina
    b. Hernial protrusion through the anterior wall of the vagina
    c. Symptoms associated with PMS
    d. Enlargement and protrusion of the cervix into the vaginal vault

12. Which finding suggests an infection with a sexually transmitted infection?
    a. Ulcers and vesicles on the vulva
    b. Atrophy of labia minora
    c. Dilation of the urethral orifice
    d. Bluish color to the cervix

13. The examiner observes a slit-shaped cervical os in a nulliparous woman. Which of the following data in her history explains this finding? The patient
    a. had an early onset of menarche.
    b. has had multiple sex partners.
    c. has had infection with the HPV.
    d. had an abortion as a teenager.

14. A prominent labia minora in a newborn
    a. indicates a maternal infection.
    b. suggests ambiguous genitalia.
    c. is consistent with prematurity.
    d. is a normal finding.

15. The mother of a 6-year-old girl expresses concern that her daughter seems to be experiencing vaginal bleeding. Which statement regarding vaginal bleeding in children is true?
    a. Vaginal bleeding in children is always a sign of sexual abuse.
    b. Vaginal bleeding in children is always clinically important.
    c. Vaginal bleeding in children is most commonly caused by carcinoma of the cervix.
    d. Occasional vaginal bleeding in the child is considered a benign finding.

16. Softness of the cervix is an expected finding for
    a. an adolescent.
    b. a pregnant woman.
    c. a nonpregnant woman.
    d. an older adult.

17. In what way is the pelvic outlet estimated on a pregnant patient?
    a. Insert a speculum into the patient's vagina and open as widely as possible. Measure the distance between the two blades.
    b. Insert two fingers into the vagina until fingers touch the cervix. Measure the distance to the cervix.
    c. Place the palm of the hand over the perineum, spread fingers to the width of the ischial tuberosities, and measure.
    d. Use a Thom pelvimeter to measure the bi-ischial diameter.

18. A cauliflower-like mass found on the labia of a female patient is most likely caused by
    a. primary syphilis.
    b. condyloma latum.
    c. condyloma acuminatum.
    d. venereal herpes.

19. A sexually active, single, 22-year-old patient complains of a "gross" vaginal discharge. Which of the following questions would help the examiner understand this symptom?
    a. "Do you use condoms?"
    b. "What type of oral contraceptives do you take?"
    c. "At what age did you start menstruating?"
    d. "Do you have a family history of ovarian or breast cancer?"

20. A 62-year-old female patient went through menopause about 14 years ago. Which statement made by this patient indicates a need for further follow-up?
    a. "I have not been sexually active for about 4 years."
    b. "My pubic hair has become very thin."
    c. "I have small amounts of vaginal bleeding a couple of times a week."
    d. "I have been taking extra calcium since I reached menopause."

113

LEARNING OBJECTIVES

After studying Chapter 19 in the textbook and completing this section of the laboratory manual, students should be able to:

1. Conduct a history related to the male genitalia.
2. Discuss examination techniques for the male genitalia.
3. Identify normal age- and condition-related variations of the male genitalia.
4. Recognize findings that deviate from expected findings.
5. Relate symptoms or clinical findings to common pathologic conditions.

TEXTBOOK REVIEW

Chapter 19: Male Genitalia (pp. 466–484)

CHAPTER OVERVIEW

This chapter describes the anatomy and physiology of the male genitalia, including a review of sexual physiology and differences in selected populations. Related health history and physical examination findings of the male genitalia are discussed. Also reviewed are abnormal physical examination findings in relation to common pathologic diagnoses.

TERMINOLOGY REVIEW

Adhesions—inflammatory bands that connect opposing serous surfaces.

Ambiguous genitalia—a newborn's genitalia are not clearly either male or female.

Balanitis—inflammation of the glans penis and prepuce.

Chordee—ventral shortening and curvature of the penis.

Circumcision—surgical removal of the prepuce.

Condyloma acuminata—genital warts caused by human papilloma virus (HPV); invades the basal layer of the epidermis, and virus penetrates through skin and causes mucosal microabrasions.

Cremasteric—reflex characterized by rising of the scrotum and testicle when the inner thigh is stroked.

Cryptorchidism—undescended testes; a scrotum that has remained small, flat, and undeveloped.

Epididymitis—inflammation of the epididymis.

Escutcheon—pattern of hair growth on the male pubis and abdomen.

Glans—expansion at the distal end of the penis by the corpus spongiosum.

Genital herpes—sexually transmitted infection caused by herpes simplex virus (HSV); most commonly caused by the HSV-2 virus.

Hernia—protrusion of a peritoneal-lined sac through some defect in the abdominal wall.

Hydrocele—fluid accumulation in the scrotum as a result of a defect in the tunica vaginalis resulting in a nontender, smooth, firm mass.

Hypospadias—congenital defect in which the urethral meatus is located on the ventral surface of the glans penile shaft or the base of the penis; congenital defect that is thought to occur embryologically during urethral development.

Klinefelter—XXY chromosomal anomaly; caused by an extra X chromosome.

Lymphogranuloma venereum—sexually transmitted infection that of the lymphatics; caused by *Chlamydia trachomatis*, which enters through skin breaks and abrasions and across as the epithelial cells of mucous membranes.

Molluscum contagiosum—viral inspection of the skin and mucous membranes considered a sexually transmitted infection in adults; caused by a poxvirus that enters the skin through small breaks in the skin barrier.

Orchitis—acute inflammation of the testis secondary to infection.

Peyronie—disease characterized by a fibrous band in the corpus cavernosum.

Phimosis or paraphimosis—the inability to replace the foreskin to its usual position after it has been attracted behind the glands.

Priapism—prolonged penile erection.

Spermatocele—benign cystic swelling on the epididymis.

114

Syphilitic chancre—skin lesion associated with primary syphilis; sexually transmitted infection caused by the bacterium *Treponema pallidum* generally occurs 2 weeks after exposure.

Testicular torsion—rotation producing ischemia of testis.

Varicocele—abnormal tortuosity and dilation of veins of the pampiniform plexus in the spermatic cord.

APPLICATION TO CLINICAL PRACTICE

Anatomy Review

Identify the structures of the male anatomy labeled on the illustration below by writing the correct term in the blank next to the corresponding letter. Use each term once.

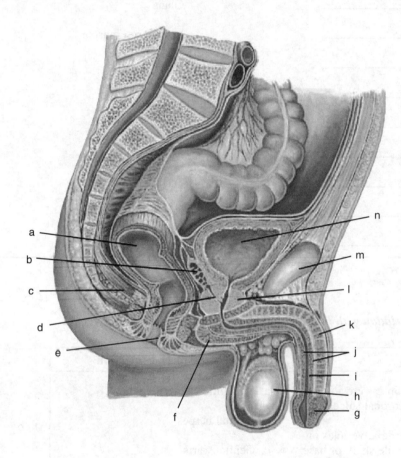

a. _____	Anus
b. _____	Bulbocavernosus muscle
c. _____	Corpus cavernosum
d. _____	Corpus spongiosum
e. _____	Ejaculatory duct
f. _____	Glans
g. _____	Levator ani muscle
h. _____	Prostate gland
i. _____	Rectum
j. _____	Seminal vesicle
k. _____	Symphysis pubis
l. _____	Testis
m. _____	Urethra
n. _____	Urinary bladder

Matching 1

Match each lesion description with the corresponding sexually transmitted infection.

Description of Lesion	Sexually Transmitted Infection
_____ 1. Initially a painless erosion on or near the coronal sulcus	a. Syphilitic chancre
_____ 2. Painful superficial vesicles on the glans, penile shaft, or base of the penis	b. Genital herpes
_____ 3. Dome-shaped, smooth, pearly gray lesions on the glans penis	c. Genital warts
_____ 4. Painless lesion with a clear base and indurated borders, usually located on the glans penis	d. Lymphogranuloma venereum
_____ 5. Reddish lesions on the prepuce, glans, and shaft; may also be present within the urethra	e. Molluscum contagiosum located on glans penis

Matching 2

Match each examination technique with its corresponding purpose.

Examination Technique	Purpose
_____ 1. Foreskin retracted	a. Inspecting for urethral discharge
_____ 2. Finger moved along vas deferens	b. Observing for hydrocele
_____ 3. Glans pressed between thumb and forefinger	c. Observing for phimosis
	d. Palpating for inguinal hernia
_____ 4. Mass transilluminated	e. Palpating for tender testes
_____ 5. Testes gently compressed	

Case Study

Mr. Corazza is a 43-year-old man who presents to the urgent care center. Listed below are data collected by the examiner.

INTERVIEW DATA

Mr. Corazza tells the examiner, "Yesterday I noticed a mild discomfort in my groin. When I looked, I saw this area of swelling." The examiner asks about recent activity. Mr. Corazza replies, "We have been in the process of moving, and I have been picking up heavy boxes, moving furniture, and climbing up and down ladders all weekend."

EXAMINATION DATA

General survey: Healthy-appearing man.

Examination: Bulge noted in area of Hesselbach triangle that is painless. Inguinal area on right side with a palpable mass. Pushes against side of finger on examination.

1. What data deviate from normal findings, suggesting a need for further investigation?

2. What additional questions could the examiner ask to clarify symptoms?

3. What additional physical examination, if any, should the examiner complete?

4. What primary problems does the patient have?

CRITICAL THINKING

1. A 30-year-old man requests information regarding self-examination of his genitalia. What information should the examiner share with him?

2. When the examiner attempts to examine the genitalia of a 5-year-old boy, the boy refuses to take off his pants and says, "You can't see my privates." What measures can the examiner take to facilitate this part of the examination?

CONTENT REVIEW QUESTIONS

Multiple Choice
Circle the correct answer for each of the following questions.

1. While examining a newborn male infant, the examiner palpates a testicle in the inguinal canal that cannot be pushed into the scrotum. This finding is consistent with
   a. hydrocele.
   b. ambiguous genitalia.
   c. direct inguinal hernia.
   d. undescended testicle.

2. The examiner is providing a 20-year-old man with information on genital self-examination (GSE). For what reason should a man this age be taught how to do this?
   a. Testicular cancer is the most common type of cancer in young men.
   b. Self-examination can help determine when full development of the genitalia is completed.
   c. Self-examination can prevent acquiring a sexually transmitted infection.
   d. Routine examination can help detect prostate enlargement.

3. The examiner has given a 20-year-old man information regarding GSE. Which statement made by the patient indicates that further teaching is necessary?
   a. "I should perform this every month on a regular schedule."
   b. "I should look for discharge or sores on my penis."
   c. "I should look for a hernia while doing this."
   d. "A good time to do this is while bathing."

4. While examining the genitalia of a 2-year-old boy, the examiner should be aware that the
   a. scrotum is normally edematous.
   b. foreskin of the uncircumcised penis is not fully retractable until age 3 or 4 years.
   c. testicles typically do not descend into the scrotum until age 5 years.
   d. the supine position is preferred for examination of children this age.

5. Which item in the patient history is considered a risk factor for cancer of the penis?
   a. Circumcised at birth
   b. History of condyloma acuminatum infections
   c. Had a congenital hydrocele
   d. History of untreated epispadias

6. In which of the following situations is transillumination of the scrotum indicated?
   a. Presence of syphilis chancre is noted.
   b. Indirect hernia is palpated.
   c. The examiner suspects a mass.
   d. The examiner palpates the testes.

7. The patient is asked to bear down while the examiner palpates the inguinal ring. The examiner feels a soft swelling sensation on the fingertip. The patient complains of pain while straining. These findings are consistent with which of the following?
   a. Indirect hernia
   b. Direct hernia
   c. Femoral hernia
   d. Rectal hernia

8. The examiner inspects the scrotum of a 43-year-old man. Which finding requires further evaluation or follow-up?
   a. The left testicle hangs lower than the right testicle.
   b. The scrotum is darker than the general skin color.
   c. The skin on the scrotum is shiny and smooth.
   d. The scrotum is divided into two sacs by a septum.

9. Which finding may indicate diabetes?
   a. The vas deferens feels beaded or lumpy.
   b. The testicle feels hard with a lump.
   c. Sebaceous cysts are present on the scrotal skin.
   d. The urethra has a slitlike orifice.

10. During an examination for a hernia, an adult male patient should
    a. be asked to stand.
    b. be in a supine position.
    c. sit on a table with the heels together.
    d. assume a knee–chest position on the examination table.

11. Balanitis associated with phimosis occurs only in
    a. newborn male infants.
    b. men with diabetes.
    c. uncircumcised men.
    d. men exposed to radiation.

12. Which of the following testicular characteristics is (are) associated with syphilis or diabetic neuropathy?
    a. Asymmetry and dropping
    b. Bilateral enlargement
    c. Insensitivity to pain
    d. Migration into the abdomen

13. What type of hernia would you most likely see in a 15-year-old young man?
    a. Femoral hernia
    b. Umbilical hernia
    c. Direct inguinal hernia
    d. Indirect inguinal hernia

14. Which of the following scrotal findings is expected for a full-term newborn boy?
    a. Fibrosis
    b. Pendulous
    c. Smooth
    d. Without rugae

15. A 24-year-old man has scrotal pain and marked erythema. The examiner considers epididymitis. Which finding is consistent with this problem?
    a. The patient's scrotal size and shape are not symmetric.
    b. The patient has anorexia and nausea.
    c. The patient reports an acute onset of severe pain.
    d. Urinalysis shows elevated WBCs and bacteria.

16. Hypospadias is a congenital defect in which the urethra meatus is located on the ventral surface of the glans penis. This is thought to occur embryologically during urethral development during which stage of gestation?
    a. 4 to 6 weeks
    b. 8 to 20 weeks
    c. 15 to 25 weeks
    d. 20 to 30 weeks

17. Which of the following hernias occurs more often in females and is the least occurring of all hernias?
    a. Indirect
    b. Direct
    c. Femoral
    d. Ventral

18. Congenital defect in which the urethral meatus is located on the ventral surface of the penis is
    a. hypophysis.
    b. phimosis.
    c. epispadias.
    d. hypospadias.

19. You examine Mr. LaCosta, a 22-year-old patient. His chief complaint is penile pain and swelling. On examination, you note a constricting band of tissue directly behind the head of the penis. You diagnose this as
    a. phimosis.
    b. hypospadias.
    c. orchitis.
    d. torsion.

20. You are examining a patient and note pearly gray, smooth, umbilicated lesions. The most common cause of these lesions is
    a. syphilis.
    b. condyloma acuminata.
    c. molluscum contagiosum.
    d. lymphogranuloma venereum.

20 Anus, Rectum, and Prostate

LEARNING OBJECTIVES

After studying Chapter 20 in the textbook and completing this section of the laboratory manual, students should be able to:
1. Conduct a history related to the anus, rectum, and prostate.
2. Discuss examination techniques for the anus, rectum, and prostate.
3. Identify normal age- and condition-related variations of the anus, rectum, and prostate.
4. Recognize findings that deviate from expected findings.
5. Relate symptoms or clinical findings to common pathologic conditions.

TEXTBOOK REVIEW

Chapter 20: Anus, Rectum, and Prostate (pp. 485–500)

CHAPTER OVERVIEW

This chapter examines the anatomy and physiology of the anus, rectum, and prostate. The anatomy of special populations is also discussed. The health history related to the anus, rectum, and prostate is reviewed, and normal and abnormal physical examination findings are evaluated. Finally, common pathologic disorders are examined and correlated to symptoms and abnormal clinical findings.

TERMINOLOGY REVIEW

Anal canal—terminal portion of the rectum; lined by columns of mucosal tissue (columns of Morgagni), that fuse to form the anorectal junction.

Anal fistula—inflammatory tract that runs from the anus or rectum and opens onto the surface of the perianal skin or other tissue; caused by inflammation from a perianal or perirectal abscess.

Anal warts (condyloma acuminata)—Growths in or around the anus and genital area, the result of an infection with the human papilloma virus.

Anorectal fissure—a tear in the anal mucosa; appears most often in the posterior midline as a result of posttraumatic passage of large hard stools.

Benign prostatic hypertrophy—benign growth of the prostate gland common in men older than 50 years of age.

Enterobiasis (roundworm or pinworm)—infection caused by a small, thin, white roundworm (*Enterobius vermicularis*) adult nematode (parasite) that lives in the rectum or colon and emerges onto the perianal skin to lay eggs while the person sleeps; common in children.

Hemorrhoids—varicose veins in the rectum that may be external below the anorectal line or internal above the anorectal line; caused by pressure on the veins in the pelvic and rectal areas from straining, diarrhea, constipation, or prolonged sitting.

Imperforate anus—a congenital defect in which the rectal opening is blocked or missing; one of a variety of anorectal malformations that can occur during fetal development.

Perianal and perirectal abscesses—infection of the soft tissues surrounding the anal canal; infections caused by anaerobic organisms, usually poly microbial.

Pilonidal cyst—a cyst or sinus near the class of the buttocks; excessive pressure or repetitive trauma to the sacrococcygeal area predisposes individuals to the development of the cyst.

Polyp—abnormal growth of tissue projecting from the mucous membrane; may occur anywhere in the intestinal tract and be malignant or benign.

Prostate gland—a gland located at the base of the bladder and surrounding the urethra; it is composed of muscular and glandular tissue.

Prostatitis—inflammation or infection of the prostate gland.

Pruritus ani—itching of the anal area; commonly caused by fungal infection in adults and by parasites in children.

Rectal prolapse—condition in which the rectal mucosa (with or without the muscular wall) protrudes through the anal ring; results from constipation, diarrhea, or sometimes severe coughing or straining.

Rectum—the terminal portion of the gastrointestinal tract.

APPLICATION TO CLINICAL PRACTICE

Anatomy Review 1

Identify the structures of the rectum labeled on the illustration by writing the correct term in the blank next to the corresponding letter.

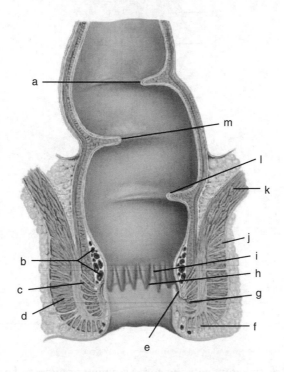

a. _____	Anal crypt
b. _____	Deep external sphincter
c. _____	Inferior rectal valve
d. _____	Internal hemorrhoidal plexus
e. _____	Internal sphincter
f. _____	Levator ani muscle
g. _____	Middle rectal valve
h. _____	Perianal gland
i. _____	Rectal column
j. _____	Rectal sinus
k. _____	Subcutaneous external sphincter
l. _____	Superficial external sphincter
m. _____	Superior rectal valve

Anatomy Review 2

Identify the structures of the prostate labeled on the illustration by writing the correct term in the blank next to the corresponding letter.

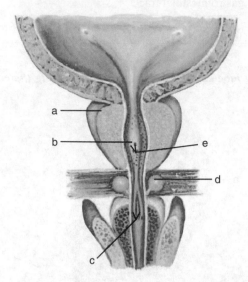

a. _____	Cowper gland
b. _____	Ejaculatory orifice
c. _____	Opening of Cowper gland
d. _____	Prostate gland
e. _____	Utricle

Matching

Match each examination finding or symptom with the corresponding problem to be considered.

Examination finding or symptom	Problem
_____ 1. Severe rectal pain with a fever	a. Prostatitis
_____ 2. Absence of meconium stool passage in an infant	b. Perianal abscess
	c. Rectal polyp
_____ 3. Feels smooth and firm with a 4-cm protrusion into the rectum	d. Benign prostatic hypertrophy with purulent drainage
_____ 4. Elevated red granular tissue opening on perianal skin	e. Prostatic carcinoma
_____ 5. Feels boggy, enlarged, and tender to palpation	f. Imperforate anus
	g. Anorectal fistula
_____ 6. Feels hard, nodular; unable to palpate sulcus	
_____ 7. Soft nodules palpated with rectal examination	

Concepts Application

Fill in the following table by comparing the different methods of screening for prostate cancer.

Screening Method	What It Reflects	What Results Mean	When It Is Indicated
DRE			
PSA			
PSA velocity			
Free PSA ratio			
Biopsy			
TRUS			

Case Study

Mr. Murphy is a 66-year-old man who presents to his primary care provider complaining of a 3-month history of rectal fullness. Listed below are data collected by the examiner during an interview and examination.

INTERVIEW DATA

Mr. Murphy tells the examiner he has had pain "off and on" but became concerned when he started seeing blood in his stool. The blood is described as "bright red." Mr. Murphy also states that he has seen spots on his underwear, but he has ignored it, thinking he had hemorrhoids. When asked about changes in his diet, Mr. Murphy indicates that he really hasn't been very hungry lately and has lost 10 pounds over the past several months.

EXAMINATION DATA

General survey: Thin-appearing man. Vital signs are within normal limits.

Rectal examination: Perineal and anal inspection is unremarkable with no lesions, dimpling, or changes in skin characteristics. Sphincter tone findings unremarkable. A large mass is felt with rectal palpation extending from the posterior to the left lateral rectal wall. The prostate is smooth, firm, and nontender to palpation with a 1-cm protrusion.

1. What data deviate from normal findings, suggesting a need for further investigation?

2. What additional questions could the examiner ask to clarify symptoms?

3. What additional physical examination, if any, should the examiner complete?

4. What primary problems does the patient have?

CRITICAL THINKING

1. A 68-year-old man comes to the emergency department with a history of urinary retention. He states, "I know my bladder is full, but I can't seem to pee." This symptom could be caused by prostatitis, benign prostate hypertrophy, or prostatic carcinoma. How does the examiner differentiate the cause of this patient's symptom?

2. A 70-year-old woman comes to a clinic with a complaint of rectal bleeding. There are multiple causes of rectal bleeding. What kind of interview questions should be asked to help the examiner narrow down the cause of the problem?

CONTENT REVIEW QUESTIONS

Multiple Choice
Circle the correct answer for each of the following questions.

1. While palpating the lateral and posterior rectal walls, the examiner should expect to palpate
   a. a smooth, even, and uninterrupted surface.
   b. small nodules from internal hemorrhoids.
   c. tissue folds from the valves of Houston.
   d. bulging from the bladder wall.

2. A patient presents with a chief complaint of rectal pain. The examiner will focus the history and examination on which known fact?
   a. Rectal pain is almost always accompanied by an infection.
   b. Rectal pain is almost always an indication of local disease.
   c. A complaint of rectal pain is usually associated with a serious systemic process.
   d. One of the most common causes of rectal pain is prostatic enlargement.

3. During an examination, the examiner observes inflammation of the sacrococcygeal area. The patient complains of pain when the area is palpated. Which of the following problems is *not* consistent with such a finding?
   a. Anorectal fistula
   b. Pilonidal cyst
   c. Hemorrhoids
   d. Perianal abscess

4. While examining the perineum of a 6-year-old girl, the examiner observes hemorrhoids. This finding suggests
   a. repeated events of sexual abuse.
   b. the presence of chronic constipation.
   c. a diet high in fibrous foods.
   d. an underlying problem such as portal hypertension.

5. To examine a prostate, what surface is palpated?
   a. Anterior rectal wall surface
   b. Posterior rectal wall surface
   c. Anterior prostate surface
   d. Deep external sphincter surface

6. A patient tells the examiner that she has had clay-colored stools. Stool of this color results from
   a. a lack of bile pigment.
   b. excessive fiber intake.
   c. excessive dietary beef.
   d. insufficient fluid intake.

7. An older male patient is unable to assume a standing position for a routine rectal examination. What is the best alternative position?
   a. Lithotomy position
   b. Left lateral position with the knees flexed
   c. Knee–chest position
   d. Prone position

8. A pregnant woman presents to the emergency department with a complaint of dark stools. She tells the examiner, "I read in a magazine that this is a sign of bleeding." Which of the following questions by the examiner is most applicable for this situation?
   a. "Where did you read that information?"
   b. "Have you been giving yourself enemas?"
   c. "How much fruit and vegetable intake have you had in the past few days?"
   d. "Are you taking prenatal vitamins?"

9. Before palpating the prostate, the examiner should tell the patient that he might feel the urge to do which of the following?
   a. Urinate
   b. Defecate
   c. Vomit
   d. Faint

10. Which of the following is considered a routine screening test done in conjunction with a rectal examination?
    a. Biopsy of rectal tissue to rule out precancerous cells
    b. Smear of rectal lining to rule out infectious disease
    c. Transillumination of the rectum to detect a mass
    d. Guaiac test of stool to rule out presence of blood

11. Which examination finding in the child is a clue to the diagnosis of Hirschsprung disease?
    a. Passing of frequent, loose stools in the absence of other symptoms
    b. Consistently empty rectum with a history of constipation
    c. Itching and irritation around the anus
    d. Rectal prolapse

12. In which situation would the examiner perform a rectal examination on an infant or child?
    a. A newborn infant passes a greenish-black, viscous stool 12 hours after birth.
    b. The mother of a 3-month-old baby describes the baby's stools as "loose and golden yellow."
    c. A stool of a 6-year-old child is guaiac positive.
    d. A mother tells the examiner that her 3-year-old child was sent home from day care after two episodes of diarrhea.

13. How is the anal ring assessed?
    a. Inspection of the anus
    b. External palpation of the anus
    c. Examination of the stool
    d. Rotation of a finger within the anal sphincter

14. Which of the following best describes the feel of a normal prostate gland?
    a. Soft olive or grape
    b. Small sea sponge
    c. Ping-pong ball
    d. Pencil eraser

15. Anal patency is verified in a newborn infant by
    a. inserting a lubricated thermometer through the anus and into the rectum.
    b. inserting the fifth digit through the anus and into the rectum.
    c. assessing for the passage of a meconium stool in the first 24 to 48 hours after birth.
    d. inspecting the anus for an anal opening.

16. Prostate enlargement is determined by the
    a. diameter of the rectum near the bladder.
    b. circumference of the prostate.
    c. estimation of the depth of the sulcus.
    d. protrusion of the prostate into the rectum.

17. Which of the following patients has a known risk factor for colorectal cancer?
    a. Marcus, a 21-year-old college student who is a vegetarian
    b. Jack, a 56-year-old man who eats a diet high in beef
    c. Susan, a 38-year-old woman with a 5-year history of gastric ulcers
    d. Helen, a 22-year-old mother with multiple hemorrhoids

18. A mother tells the examiner that her 2-year-old son has an odd, bright red bulge coming out of his anus that "looks like a donut." What kind of problem does this history suggest?
    a. Pin worms
    b. Pilonidal cyst
    c. Rectal prolapse
    d. Hypertrophy of the anus

19. The examiner palpates a prostate, noting that it is hard and irregular. The median sulcus is not palpable. These findings are consistent with
    a. prostate cancer.
    b. benign prostatic hypertrophy.
    c. prostatitis.
    d. rectal mass.

20. A rectal prolapse in a young child is frequently associated with
    a. rickets.
    b. cystic fibrosis.
    c. Crohn disease.
    d. chronic constipation or diarrhea.

21 Musculoskeletal System

LEARNING OBJECTIVES

After studying Chapter 21 in the textbook and completing this section of the laboratory manual, students should be able to:
1. Conduct a history related to the musculoskeletal system.
2. Discuss examination techniques for the musculoskeletal system.
3. Identify normal age- and condition-related variations of the musculoskeletal system.
4. Recognize findings that deviate from expected findings.
5. Relate symptoms or clinical findings to common pathologic conditions.

TEXTBOOK REVIEW

Chapter 21: Musculoskeletal System (pp. 501–543)

CHAPTER OVERVIEW

This chapter reviews the anatomy and physiology of the musculoskeletal system, including variations of special populations. Interviewing techniques effective in gathering information about the musculoskeletal system are discussed, as well as techniques for physical examination. Health history and physical examination findings that deviate from normal are evaluated to correlate with clinical findings of common pathologic conditions of the musculoskeletal system, which provides for the stability and mobility necessary for physical activity.

TERMINOLOGY REVIEW

Abduction—movement of the extremities away from the body.

Adduction—movement of the extremities toward the body.

Ankylosing spondylitis—a hereditary chronic inflammatory disease; may affect the cervical, thoracic, and lumbar sign and also involves the sacroiliac joints; leads to eventual fusion and severe deformity of the vertebral column.

Bursitis—inflammation of the bursa caused by repetitive movement and excessive pressure on the bursa.

Carpal tunnel syndrome—compression on the median nerve at the wrist within its flexor tendon sheath caused by microtrauma, local edema, repetitive motion, or vibration of the hands.

Claw toe—hyperextension of the metatarsophalangeal joint with flexion of the toe's proximal and distal joints.

Clubfoot—a fixed congenital defect of the ankle and foot.

Crepitus—crackling sound heard in the patient's joint with movement.

Dislocation—complete separation of the contact between two bones in a joint; caused by pressure or force pushing the bone out of the joint; usually occurs in the setting of acute trauma.

Dupuytren contracture—contractures involving the flexor hand tendons; flexor tendons generally of the fourth and fifth digits contract, causing the fingers to curl with impaired extension.

Eversion—movement of the sole of the foot outward at the ankle.

Fracture—a partial or complete break in the continuity of a bone.

Fibromyalgia—a painful nonarticular condition that leads to diffuse musculoskeletal discomfort.

Gibbus—a sharp, angular deformity associated with a collapsed vertebra caused by osteoporosis.

Goniometer—a calibrated device designed to measure the arc or range of motion (ROM) of a joint.

Gout—a form of arthritis; a disorder of purine metabolism that results from elevated serum uric acid level; monosodium urate crystal deposition enjoins and surrounding tissues, resulting in acute inflammatory attacks.

Gower sign—a sign that indicates generalized muscle weakness in children.

Hallux valgus—a deformity marked by lateral deviation of the great toe with overlapping of the second toe.

Inversion—movement of the sole of the foot inward at the ankle.

Kyphosis—outward curvature of the thoracic spine.

Legg-Calvé-Perthes disease—avascular necrosis of the femoral head; results from decreased blood supply to the femoral head.

Lordosis—concave curvature of the lumbar spine.

Lumbar stenosis—a narrowing of the spinal canal caused by hypertrophy of the ligamentum flavum and facet joints, leading to entrapment of the spinal cord as it traverses the spinal canal.

Lumbosacral radiculopathy—herniation of a lumbar disk that irritates the corresponding nerve root.

Mallet toe—a flexion deformity at the distal interphalangeal joint of the foot.

Metatarsus adductus—the most common congenital foot deformity, marked by the middle bones of the foot pointing in toward the body; can be either fixed or flexible.

Muscular dystrophy—a group of genetic disorders involving gradual degeneration of the muscle fibers.

Muscle strain—excessive stretching or forceful contraction of a muscle beyond its functional capacity.

Osgood-Schlatter disease—painful swelling of the knee caused by apophyseal traction of the anterior aspect of the tibial tubercle; common overuse injury in adolescents.

Osteoarthritis—deterioration of the articular cartilage covering the ends of bone in the synovial joints.

Osteomyelitis—an infection in the bone that usually results from an open wound or systemic infection.

Osteoporosis—decrease in bone mass that occurs when bone resorption is more rapid than bone deposition; as a result of cartilage abrasion, pitting, and thinning, the bone surfaces are eventually exposed with eventual bone rubbing against bone.

Paget disease (osteitis deformans)—a focal metabolic disorder of the bone; appears in persons older than 45 years; caused by excessive bone resorption and bone formation, producing a mosaic pattern in the lamellar bone.

Pes cavus—condition marked by a high arch on the sole of the foot.

Pes planus—condition marked by a collapsed arch of the foot; commonly called "flat foot" or "fallen arches."

Polydactyly—the presence of more than five digits on the hand or foot.

Pronation—position of the forearm so that the palm faces down; position of the heel so that the foot does not bear weight through the midline.

Radial head subluxation (nursemaid's elbow)—a dislocation injury of the elbow.

Rheumatoid arthritis (RA)—a chronic systemic inflammatory disorder of the synovial tissue surrounding the joints; polymorphonuclear leukocytes aggregate in the inflamed synovial tissue and fluid.

Rotator cuff tear—microtrauma and tearing of the rotator cuff muscles, most often the supraspinatus; usually caused by degeneration of the muscle and tendon from repeated overhead lifting.

Scoliosis—a condition marked by an abnormal curvature of the spine; the spine may look more like an S or a C.

Simian—referring to a single crease extending across the entire palm; associated with Down syndrome.

Slipped capital femoral epiphysis—a disorder in which the capital femoral epiphysis slips over the neck of the femur.

Supination—position of the forearm so that the palm faces upward.

Syndactyly—congenital fusion of the digits of the hand or foot.

Temporomandibular joint syndrome—a condition characterized by painful jaw movement; caused by congenital anomalies, malocclusion, trauma, arthritis, and other joint diseases.

Tenosynovitis—inflammation of the synovium-lined sheath around a tendon; seen with repetitive actions associated with occupational or sports activities.

Matching 1

Match each examination technique with the problem or condition it is used to detect. Some answers may be used more than once.

Examination Technique	Possible Problem or Condition
_____ 1. McMurray test	a. Anterior cruciate ligament injury
_____ 2. Ballottement	b. Effusion of fluid in the knee
_____ 3. Barlow-Ortolani maneuver	c. Flexion contractures in the hip
_____ 4. Bulge sign	d. L1, L2, L3, L4 nerve root irritation
_____ 5. Drawer test	e. Torn meniscus in knee
_____ 6. Femoral stretch test	f. Anteroposterior instability in knee
_____ 7. Lachman test	g. Mediolateral instability of knee
_____ 8. McMurray test	
_____ 9. Thomas test	
_____10. Varus/valgus stress test	

Concepts Application 1

Based on the symptoms and/or examination findings provided, list the corresponding problem(s) to consider.

Symptoms or Assessment Findings	Problems to Consider
Heberden nodes and Bouchard nodes noted on the hands	
Low back pain that radiates to the buttocks and posterior thigh with tenderness over the spine	
Heat, redness, swelling, and tenderness to the metatarsophalangeal joint	
Subcutaneous nodules on the forearm near the elbow	
Tenderness, swelling, and boggy sensation with palpation along the grooves of the olecranon process; increased pain with pronation and supination	
A child with muscle atrophy and symptoms of progressive muscle weakness	
A child complaining of pain in the elbow and wrist; will not move his or her arm; maintains arm in a flexed and pronated position	

Matching 2

Match each set of clinical findings with its corresponding diagnosis.

Clinical Findings	Diagnosis
_____ 1. Chronic inflammatory disease involving the spine and sacroiliac joints	a. Bursitis
	b. Carpal tunnel syndrome
_____ 2. Numbness, burning, and tingling in the hands	
	c. Paget disease
_____ 3. Unilateral facial pain that worsens with joint movement	d. Fibromyalgia
	e. Legg-Calvé-Perthes disease
_____ 4. Sudden onset of hot, swollen joint(s), limited ROM	f. Ankylosing spondylitis
_____ 5. Excessive bone resorption and bone formation	g. Temporomandibular joint syndrome
_____ 6. Painful, nonarticular musculoskeletal condition	h. Gout
_____ 7. Inflammation of this structure adjacent to a joint leads to limitation with motion, point tenderness, and swelling	
_____ 8. Avascular necrosis of the femoral head	

Case Study

Mrs. Simmons is a 46-year-old woman with RA. Listed below are data collected by the examiner during an interview and examination.

INTERVIEW DATA

According to the medical record, Mrs. Simmons was diagnosed with RA at the age of 30 years. She describes a great deal of pain in her joints, particularly in her hands, and says she has just learned to live with the pain because it will always be there. She states that the stiffness and pain in her joints are always worse in the morning or any time she sits around too much. She denies muscle weakness other than the fact that her stiffness and soreness prevent her from doing much. Mrs. Simmons states that the RA is progressing to the point where she is having difficulty doing things that require fine motor dexterity, such as changing clothes, holding utensils to eat, and cutting up her food. She says she can still get cleaned up but that she had to have different faucet handles installed in her home so she could turn the water on and off. Mrs. Simmons says she rarely goes out because she feels ugly.

EXAMINATION DATA

Patient is able to stand, but standing up straight and erect is not possible. Gait is slow and purposeful, with jerky movements. Significant inflammation, swelling, and tenderness are noted with inspection and palpation at the hip, knee, wrists, hands, and feet bilaterally. Subcutaneous nodules are noted at ulnar surface of elbows bilaterally.

1. What data deviate from normal findings, suggesting a need for further investigation?

2. What additional questions could the examiner ask to clarify symptoms?

3. What additional physical examination, if any, should the examiner complete?

4. What primary problems does the patient have?

CRITICAL THINKING

1. Mark is a 17-year-old young man who presents with pain in the ankle. He says he twisted it during his soccer game earlier in the afternoon, and now the pain seems to be getting worse. The ankle is very swollen with a bluish discoloration. How can the examiner determine whether Mark has a muscle strain, a sprain, or a fracture?

2. A 2-year-old girl with a dislocation of the radial head is brought to the clinic by her parents. What type of activities could cause such an injury, and what type of teaching should be provided to the parents?

CONTENT REVIEW QUESTIONS

Multiple Choice

Circle the correct answer for each of the following questions.

1. The spine of a newborn infant should be palpated with the examiner noting the shape of each spinal process. If a split is noted in one of the spinal processes, which problem is suspected?
   a. Bifid defect
   b. Lordosis
   c. Down syndrome
   d. Spina bifida

2. Which of the following questions asked by the examiner would be most helpful in understanding a patient complaining of acute back pain?
   a. "What medications do you currently take?"
   b. "Was there any activity or injury that occurred before the onset of the pain?"
   c. "Were you born with any congenital deformities of the spine?"
   d. "Have you recently lost weight?"

3. Which spinal finding would be considered normal for a 72-year-old patient?
   a. Meningocele
   b. Myelomeningocele
   c. Kyphosis
   d. Scoliosis

4. Which of the following data from a patient's history indicates an increased risk for osteomyelitis?
   a. Severe gout
   b. RA
   c. Severe osteoporosis
   d. Open fracture of the radius

5. What degree of knee flexion is considered a normal finding?
   a. 15
   b. 90
   c. 130
   d. 160

6. Which of the following is considered a normal finding for a woman in her eighth month of pregnancy?
   a. Stronger ligaments and spinal joints
   b. Hypercalcemia
   c. A 25% loss of muscle strength
   d. Lordosis

7. When assessing for carpal tunnel syndrome, the Tinel sign can be performed by tapping the
   a. dorsal aspect of the wrist.
   b. volar carpal ligament.
   c. radial artery.
   d. median nerve.

8. Which group is susceptible to subluxation of the head of the radius?
   a. Infants and toddlers
   b. Adolescents
   c. Pregnant women
   d. Older adults

9. The extension of the patient's head against the examiner's hand is a test of
   a. cervical spine alignment.
   b. passive ROM.
   c. temporalis muscle strength.
   d. sternocleidomastoid muscle strength.

10. A patient complains of pain and a clicking noise with jaw movement. The pain extends into the face. These symptoms are suggestive of what condition?
    a. Gout in the jaw
    b. Temporomandibular joint syndrome
    c. RA of the jaw
    d. Bursitis of the temporomandibular joint

11. "Normal" muscle strength is documented as grade
    a. 0.
    b. 1.
    c. 5.
    d. 10.

12. To assess muscle strength of the temporalis and masseter muscles, the examiner will ask the patient to
    a. push the jaw forward while the examiner applies counterforce.
    b. attempt to open the mouth while the examiner applies counterforce.
    c. clench the teeth while the examiner palpates the contracted muscles.
    d. clench the teeth together while the examiner attempts to open the mouth with a tongue blade.

13. For which type of problem does a family history have significance?
    a. Ankylosing spondylitis
    b. Dislocation of radius
    c. Lumbosacral radiculopathy
    d. Bursitis

14. Which statement made by a patient helps the examiner differentiate osteoarthritis from RA?
    a. "I have swelling and pain in my joints."
    b. "I notice a crackling sound when I move my joints."
    c. "I get extremely tired by mid-morning, even when I sleep well."
    d. "I used to play the piano when I was younger."

15. Which of the following would be assessed as part of ROM during the assessment of the thoracic and lumbar spine?
    a. Extend, flex, and rotate
    b. Evert, inversion, and rotation
    c. Adduct and abduct
    d. Extend, flex, and supinate

16. Mr. Manns is a 48-year-old patient who presents for the examination of his knee. On examination, you note excessive hyperextension of his knee. This may indicate
    a. genu valgum.
    b. weakness in the quadriceps muscle.
    c. weakness in the cruciate ligament.
    d. weakness in the collateral ligament.

17. A lateral curvature of the thoracic spine indicates
    a. gibbus.
    b. convex curves.
    c. lordosis.
    d. scoliosis.

18. Which of the following tests would detect a torn meniscus?
    a. Ballottement
    b. Varus stress
    c. McMurray
    d. Bulge sign

19. Mrs. Woods is a 28-year-old patient who is pregnant in her last trimester and presents to your office with complaints of numbness in her left hand. You diagnose her with carpel tunnel sydrome most likely related to
    a. repetitive movement.
    b. fluid retention.
    c. postural changes in the neck caused by pregnancy.
    d. eclampsia.

20. Mr. Davids presents to the office for a follow-up because of RA. When you ask him to explain his fatigue because of the RA, his response would be
    a. it is severe with the onset at 4 to 5 hours after rising.
    b. it is usually several hours after lunch.
    c. it occurs within 1 hour of taking his meloxicam.
    d. it occurs immediately upon rising.

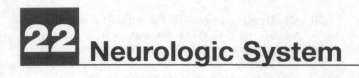

22 Neurologic System

After studying Chapter 22 in the textbook and completing this section of the laboratory manual, students should be able to:

1. Conduct a history related to the neurologic system.
2. Discuss examination techniques for the neurologic system.
3. Identify normal age- and condition-related variations of the neurologic system.
4. Recognize findings that deviate from expected findings.
5. Relate symptoms or clinical findings to common pathologic conditions.

TEXTBOOK REVIEW

Chapter 22: Neurologic System (pp. 544–580)

CHAPTER OVERVIEW

This chapter begins with a description of the anatomy and physiology of the neurologic system. Variations of the neurologic system in selected populations are also described. The interviewing techniques for a health history are reviewed, with emphasis on special populations and abnormal conditions. The evaluation of motor, sensory, autonomic, cognitive, and behavioral elements makes neurologic assessment one of the most complex portions of the physical examination. Techniques of the physical examination and recognition of abnormal findings are discussed. Finally, common pathologic disorders are described along with related symptoms and clinical findings.

TERMINOLOGY REVIEW

Antalgic—referring to behavior used to limit pain; for example, limping to reduce the time of weight bearing on an affected leg.

Ataxia—inability to coordinate muscle activity during voluntary movement.

Basal ganglia—pathway and processing station between the cerebral motor cortex and the upper brainstem.

Bell palsy—temporary acute paralysis or weakness of one side of the face.

Brainstem—pathway between the cerebral cortex and spinal cord.

Brudzinski sign—a sign characterized by involuntary flexion of the hips and knees when the neck is flexed.

Cerebellum—works with the motor cortex of the cerebrum; involved in voluntary movement; processes information from eyes, ears, and touch.

Cerebral palsy—a group of permanent disorders of movement and posture development associated with nonprogressive (static) disturbances that occurred in the developing brain of the fetus or infant.

Encephalitis—acute inflammation of the brain and spinal cord; involves the meninges and is often caused by a virus, such as transmitted by the bite of arthropod or mosquito or herpes simplex virus.

Frontal lobe—portion of the brain that contains the motor cortex; associated with voluntary skeletal movement.

Graphesthesia—tactual ability to recognize writing on the skin.

Guillain-Barré syndrome—a postinfectious disorder that occurs after a nonspecific gastrointestinal or respiratory infection that causes an acute neuromuscular paralysis.

Hypothalamus—part of the brain that maintains temperature control, water metabolism, and neuroendocrine activity.

Kernig sign—a sign assessed by flexing the leg at the knee and hip and then attempting to straighten the leg of a supine patient.

Intrapartum maternal lumbosacral plexopathy—neuropathy that can occur during late pregnancy and delivery when the lumbosacral trunk and sometimes the superior gluteal and obturator nerves are compressed between the pelvic rim and the fetal head.

Lower motor neuron disorder—absence of deep tendon reflexes may be an indication of this type of neuron disorder or of peripheral neuropathy.

Medulla oblongata—base or hindmost part of the brain; acts as the respiratory center and relay center for major ascending and descending spinal tracts.

Meningitis—inflammation of the meninges, the membranes around the brain and spinal cord; a bacterial, viral, or fungal organism often colonizes in the upper respiratory tract, invades the bloodstream, and then crosses the blood–brain barrier to infect the cerebrospinal fluid and meninges.

Multiple sclerosis—a progressive autoimmune disorder characterized by a combination of inflammation and degeneration of the myelin sheath of the brain's white matter, leading to decreased brain mass and obstruction of the transmission of nerve impulses; it has a gradual but unpredictable progression.

Myasthenia gravis—an autoimmune disorder of neuromuscular junction involved with muscle activation; autoantibodies directed against the acetylcholine receptors in the neuromuscular junction cause destruction and inflammatory changes in the postsynaptic membranes that lead to muscle dysfunction.

Myelomeningocele (spina bifida)—a congenital vertebral defect (commonly at the lumbar or sacral level) that allows the spinal cord contents to protrude.

Normal-pressure hydrocephalus—a syndrome simulating degenerative disease that is caused by noncommunicating hydrocephalus (dilated ventricles with intracranial pressure within expected ranges).

Nuchal rigidity—stiff neck; associated with meningitis.

Occipital lobe—portion of the brain that contains the primary visual center and is involved in the interpretation of visual data.

Parkinson disease—a slowly progressive, degenerative neurologic disorder associated with a deficiency of the dopamine neurotransmitter that results in poor communication between parts of the brain that coordinate and control movement and balance.

Peripheral neuropathy—a disorder of the peripheral nervous system that results in motor and sensory loss in the distribution of one or more nerves commonly caused by diabetes mellitus.

Postpolio syndrome (progressive postpoliomyelitis muscular atrophy)—the reappearance of neurologic signs 10 or more years after survival of acute poliomyelitis.

Pseudotumor cerebri—a clinical syndrome of intracranial hypertension that mimics brain tumors; potential causes include use of certain medications or metabolic, infections, or hematologic causes.

Romberg sign—a sign assessed as positive when a patient standing with eyes closed is unable to maintain balance.

Seizure disorder (epilepsy)—a chronic disorder characterized by recurrent, unprovoked seizures secondary to an underlying brain abnormality.

Shaken baby syndrome—a severe form of child abuse resulting from the violent shaking of infants younger than 1 year of age.

Steppage gait—an unexpected gait pattern manifested by an excessive lift of the hip and knee and an inability to walk on the heels.

Stereognosis—ability to identify an object by touch.

Stroke [brain attack or cerebrovascular accident (CVA)]—sudden interruption in the blood supply to a part of the brain or by the rupture of a blood vessel; two types: ischemic or hemorrhagic stroke.

Temporal lobe—portion of the brain responsible for perception and balance, as well as interpretation of sounds, tastes, and smells.

Thalamus—part of the brain that conveys sensory impulses to and from the cerebrum and integrates the impulses between the motor cortex and the cerebrum.

Trigeminal neuralgia (tic douloureux)—recurrent paroxysmal sharp pain that radiates into one or more branches of the fifth cranial nerve.

Anatomy Review 1

Identify the structures of the skull and brain labeled on the illustration by writing the correct term in the blank next to the corresponding letter.

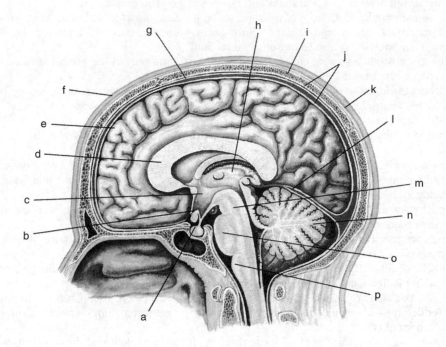

a. _____   Cerebellum

b. _____   Cerebrum

c. _____   Corpus callosum

d. _____   Dura mater (two layers)

e. _____   Galea aponeurotica

f. _____   Hypothalamus

g. _____   Medulla oblongata

h. _____   Midbrain

i. _____   Optic chiasma

j. _____   Pituitary gland

k. _____   Pons

l. _____   Skin

m. _____   Skull

n. _____   Superior sagittal sinus

o. _____   Tentorium cerebelli

p. _____   Thalamus

Anatomy Review 2

Identify the cranial nerves or structures of the skull and brain labeled on the illustration by writing the correct term in the blank next to the corresponding letter.

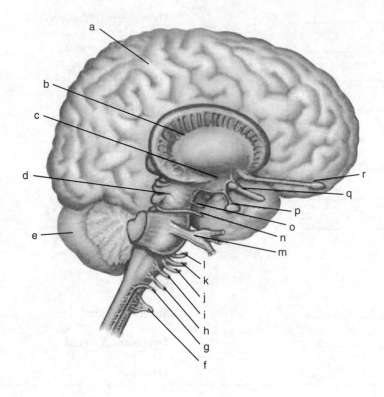

a. _____   Abducens (VI)

b. _____   Acoustic (VIII)

c. _____   Cerebellum

d. _____   Cerebral peduncle

e. _____   Cerebrum

f. _____   Facial (VII)

g. _____   Glossopharyngeal (IX)

h. _____   Hypoglossal (XII)

i. _____   Hypothalamus

j. _____   Oculomotor (III)

k. _____   Olfactory (I)

l. _____   Optic (II)

m. _____   Pituitary gland

n. _____   Spinal accessory (XI)

o. _____   Thalamus

p. _____   Trigeminal (IV)

q. _____   Trochlear (IV)

r. _____   Vagus (X)

Concepts Application 1

Complete the following table by listing the cranial nerve(s) tested by each examination procedure. More than one cranial nerve may be tested by each procedure.

Examination Procedure	Cranial Nerve(s) Tested
Whisper test	
Patient sticks out tongue and moves it from side to side	
Taste test with sugar, salt, and lemon	
Visual acuity	
Patient puffs out cheeks and shows teeth	
Patient shrugs shoulders against examiner's hands	
Smell test with coffee, orange, and cloves	
Eyes constrict and dilate in response to light	
Patient clenches teeth (temporal muscles contracted)	

Concepts Application 2

In the table below, write the name of the reflex based on the observed response; then indicate whether this reflex is expected or unexpected based on the age of the infant and/or the nature of the response.

Age of Infant	Observed Response	Name of Reflex	Expected or Unexpected?
2 months	The infant demonstrates a strong grasp of the examiner's finger when it is placed in the infant's palm.		
4 months	When held in an upright position with the soles of the feet touching the surface of a table, the infant flexes the legs upward in a curled position and holds them there.		
6 months	With the child lying supine, turn the head to one side; the arm and leg extend on the side the head was turned toward.		
8 months	The infant abducts and extends the arms and legs in response to sudden movement of the head and trunk backward. The arms then adduct in an embracing motion followed by relaxation.		

Matching

Match each set of characteristic findings with its corresponding diagnosis.

Characteristic Findings	Diagnosis
_____ 1. Fatigue, bowel and bladder dysfunction, sexual dysfunction, sensory changes, muscle weakness	a. Myasthenia gravis
	b. Generalized seizure disorder
_____ 2. A chronic disorder characterized by recurrent, unprovoked disturbances in consciousness, behavior, sensation, and autonomic functioning secondary to an underlying brain abnormality	c. Multiple sclerosis
	d. Trigeminal neuralgia
	e. Cerebral vascular accident
_____ 3. Fever, chills, headache, and nuchal rigidity	f. Cerebral palsy
	g. Meningitis
_____ 4. Sudden weakness and numbness; confusion; difficulty speaking; loss of balance; paralysis of face, arm, or leg	h. Guillain-Barré syndrome
	i. Parkinson disease
_____ 5. An autoimmune disorder of neuromuscular junction involved with muscle activation	
_____ 6. Progressive bilateral and symmetric distal weakness, diminished reflexes in ascending pattern, difficulty walking	
_____ 7. Recurrent paroxysmal sharp pain that radiates onto cranial nerve V	
_____ 8. Static and nonprogressive cerebral lesions that cause significant motor delay in a child	
_____ 9. Progressive, degenerative neurologic disorder in older adults	

Case Study

Melvin Thomas is a 64-year-old man admitted to the hospital with a diagnosis of acute CVA. Listed below are data collected by the examiner during an interview and examination.

INTERVIEW DATA

Mr. Thomas's wife tells the examiner that her husband was fine until this morning when he suddenly had a headache, fell to the floor, and could not get up. Mrs. Thomas adds that when she tried to get her husband to speak, he made only mumbling noises, and she could not understand him.

EXAMINATION DATA

Mental status: Awake, alert man. Unable to talk but able to follow commands. Very distraught over this incident. Patient cries and avoids eye contact with his wife and the examiner.

Neurologic examination: Cranial nerves I, II, III, IV, V, VI, and VII all intact. Patient has asymmetry and unequal movements of his face, with a drooping of the left side of his face. Has asymmetry of shoulder shrug, with deficiency noted on the left side. Patient has left-sided paralysis. Demonstrates expected muscle tone and sensation on right side. Unable to assess balance. Patient unable to get up or move around in bed unassisted at this time.

1. What data deviate from normal findings, suggesting a need for further investigation?

2. What additional questions could the examiner ask to clarify symptoms?

3. What additional physical examination, if any, should the examiner complete?

4. What primary problems does the patient have?

CRITICAL THINKING

1. Kevin, an ambitious novice examiner, uses an unfolded paper clip to test peripheral two-point discrimination. He adjusts the paper clip so that the points are 1 inch apart. With this instrument, he tests the patient's palm, toe, back, upper arm, and upper leg, He notes that the patient fails to discriminate between one and two points in each of these areas. Kevin concludes that the patient has some sort of peripheral sensory deficit. What is incorrect in Kevin's methods or conclusion?

2. The computed tomography scan of a patient demonstrates an infarction of the frontal lobe toward the left side. What brain functions occur in the frontal lobe? What type of symptoms would you anticipate this patient to have?

Multiple Choice

Circle the correct answer for each of the following questions.

1. Which of the following disorders is known to be hereditary?
   a. Peripheral neuropathy
   b. Meningitis
   c. Huntington chorea
   d. Seizure disorder

2. Which cranial nerve is not routinely tested unless a problem is suspected?
   a. I
   b. II
   c. V
   d. XI

3. The patient is able to touch each finger to his thumb in rapid sequence. What does this finding mean? The patient has
   a. intact trochlear and abducens cranial nerves.
   b. appropriate cerebellar function.
   c. an intact spinal accessory nerve.
   d. appropriate kinesthetic sensation.

4. Which question asked by the examiner may help determine prevention strategies for seizures that a patient has been experiencing?
   a. "Where do your seizures typically begin?"
   b. "How do you feel after the seizure?"
   c. "What goes through your mind during the seizure?"
   d. "Are there any factors or activities that seem to start the seizures?"

5. A patient makes the following statement: "I sometimes feel as if the whole room is spinning." What type of neurologic dysfunction should the examiner suspect?
   a. Peripheral neuropathy dysfunction
   b. Increased intracranial pressure from a brain tumor
   c. Inner ear dysfunction affecting the acoustic nerve
   d. Lesion affecting the frontal lobe

6. The examiner asks the patient to close her eyes and then places a vibrating tuning fork on the patient's ankle and asks her to indicate what is felt. What is being assessed?
   a. Peripheral nerve sensory function
   b. Cranial nerve sensory function
   c. Primary sensory function
   d. Level of consciousness

7. Sensory neurologic testing is not usually done with children until they are
   a. preschool age.
   b. kindergarten age.
   c. middle school age.
   d. high school age.

8. Jack is a 52-year-old obese man with a history of poorly controlled diabetes. He also smokes. Based on these data, the examiner should recognize that Jack has several risk factors for
   a. seizures.
   b. CVA.
   c. multiple sclerosis.
   d. Guillain-Barré syndrome.

9. Which of the following assessment findings should not be surprising to an examiner given Jack's history as described in question 8?
   a. Inability to discern superficial touch or two-point discrimination on the legs
   b. Reduced muscle tone on left side of the face
   c. Asymmetry of the face when asked to smile and puff out his cheeks
   d. Slow and uncoordinated movement with the finger–nose test

10. The examiner is assessing deep tendon reflex response in a 12-year-old boy. The boy's response is an expected reflex. Which of the following scores should be documented?
    a. 1+
    b. 2+
    c. 3+
    d. 4+

11. An older patient tells the examiner, "I have a hard time finding the right words when I am talking." This symptom may be
    a. a precursor to a seizure disorder.
    b. an early symptom of Parkinson disease.
    c. an indication of a dysfunction of the temporal lobe.
    d. associated with a problem of the vestibular apparatus.

12. What response should occur when a patient's field of gaze moves from a distant object to one close to his or her face?
    a. Rapid eye movement
    b. Ptosis of the eye
    c. Constriction of the pupil
    d. Dilation of the iris

13. How can an examiner best gain the cooperation of a child to perform a neurologic examination?
    a. Ask a parent to perform the examination while the examiner observes the response.
    b. Ask the mother or father to step out of the room.
    c. Promise the child a toy or treat if he or she does what you ask.
    d. Create a game from various aspects of the neurologic examination.

14. Which of the following infant reflex responses is considered normal?
    a. A 13-month-old baby's toes fan in response to stroking the lateral surface of the infant's sole.
    b. An 8-month-old infant demonstrates a positive Moro reflex when startled.
    c. A 3-month-old infant's fingers fan when the examiner's finger is placed in the infant's hand.
    d. A 2-month-old infant's legs flex up against the body when the infant is held in an upright position, and the dorsal side of the foot touches the table.

15. The examiner is conducting an interview with the mother of an infant as part of the neurologic system examination. Which of the following responses made by the mother may indicate a need for further evaluation?
    a. "My baby sometimes falls asleep when I am feeding her."
    b. "My baby seems to jump when there is a loud noise in the room."
    c. "I drank a glass of wine about once a week while I was pregnant."
    d. "I had problems with hypertension the entire time I was pregnant."

16. A patient demonstrates impaired pain sensation. Which additional test is appropriate to further evaluate this finding?
    a. Heat and cold sensation
    b. Ultrasonic perception
    c. Deep tendon reflex
    d. Transillumination of the involved area

17. The examiner squeezes the patient's biceps muscle as part of an examination. Which of the following responses verbalized by the patient is considered normal?
    a. "That makes my arm tingle."
    b. "That makes a burning sensation go up my arm."
    c. "That is uncomfortable."
    d. "My arm is twitching."

18. Which of the following findings is associated with an increased risk for skin breakdown and injury?
    a. Inability to feel pressure applied by a monofilament
    b. Inability to identify a familiar object by touch
    c. Inability to identify a letter drawn in the palm of the hand
    d. 3+ deep tendon reflexes

19. Mrs. Sanders had a CVA 2 days ago. She moves when her name is called, and she moans when she experiences painful stimuli. Which of the following best describes Mrs. Sanders' level of consciousness?
    a. Confusion
    b. Delirium
    c. Lethargy
    d. Stupor

20. Mr. Stanton is a 52-year-old patient with diabetes who presents to the office for a routine examination. You have checked protective sensation with 5.07 monofilament, and you noted a loss of sensation. This indicates
    a. peripheral neuropathy.
    b. positive Kernig sign.
    c. positive Brudzinski sign.
    d. posturing.

23 Sports Participation Evaluation

LEARNING OBJECTIVES

After studying Chapter 23 in the textbook and completing this section of the laboratory manual, students should be able to:
1. Describe health history and physical examination techniques for the participation examination.
2. Discuss the required components of the preparticipation examination.
3. Describe a 14-step musculoskeletal examination.
4. Review pathologic conditions and determination for sports participation.

TEXTBOOK REVIEW

Chapter 23: Sports Participation Evaluation (pp. 581–593)

CHAPTER OVERVIEW

This chapter examines the health history and physical examination techniques required for the sports participation evaluation. Recommended components of the preparticipation examination are discussed in detail. Various pathologic conditions are described, with a focus on the related ability to participate in a specific sport. The musculoskeletal component of the preparticipation examination is highlighted.

TERMINOLOGY REVIEW

Atlantoaxial instability—condition in which the joint is excessively mobile; there may be no neurologic complications at first, but risk exists for subluxation and spinal cord compression.
Female athlete triad—a trio of problems including disordered eating, amenorrhea, and osteoporosis.
Oligomenorrhea—interval between periods greater than 35 days.
Primary amenorrhea—no onset of menses by 16 years of age.
Sports-related concussion—a complex pathophysiologic process affecting the brain induced by traumatic biomechanical forces.

APPLICATION TO CLINICAL PRACTICE

For each component of the preparticipation examination listed, identify the specific recommended elements (data to obtain, assessments to complete).

Examination Component	Recommended Elements of Examination
Medical history	
Cardiac	
Respiratory	
Neurologic	
Vision	
Orthopedic	
Psychosocial	
Genitourinary	

CRITICAL THINKING

1. Emilio Sanchez is a 17-year-old adolescent who presents for a preparticipation examination for wrestling. On examination, his blood pressure is 126/82 mm Hg. His height is 5'9" (50th percentile for age), and his weight is 65 kg (50th percentile for age). His blood pressure at his last visit 1 year ago was 110/70 mm Hg. He is asymptomatic today.
   a. How should his hypertension be classified?

   b. What are the next steps in evaluating his elevated blood pressure?

   c. What classification of contact is wrestling?

   d. Which components of the preparticipation examination should be completed?

2. David Rose is an 18-year-old senior high school football player who presents after having experienced a concussion during a game 4 days ago. His father reports that David lost consciousness for about 2 minutes. He has been having headaches, but he is eager to get back to football practice.
   a. What type of concussion did David experience?

   b. What are the next steps in his evaluation?

Multiple Choice

Circle the correct answer for each of the following questions.

1. The main purpose in determining the normal neuro-psychologic status in the preparticipation examination is to
   a. clear the individual for all sports participation.
   b. allow you to better judge the return to normal in the event of injury.
   c. judge the ability for the individual to play contact sports.
   d. ensure that subsequent preparticipation examinations can be brief.

2. During the preparticipation examination, the component that detects problems affecting the athlete is the
   a. neurologic evaluation.
   b. musculoskeletal examination.
   c. history.
   d. general physical examination.

3. The female athlete triad includes
   a. eating disorder, amenorrhea, and osteoporosis.
   b. thyroid dysfunction, eating disorder, and amenorrhea.
   c. stress fractures, thyroid dysfunction, and oligo-menorrhea.
   d. eating disorder, thyroid dysfunction, and osteoporosis.

4. In female athletes during teenage years, an overly thin body frame encourages
   a. primary amenorrhea.
   b. thyroid dysfunction.
   c. an eating disorder.
   d. a hypoestrogenic state.

5. Mary Simmons is an 18-year-old developmentally dis-abled patient with a history of hypothyroidism, bipolar disorder, allergies, and asthma. She is requesting a pre-participation examination for the Special Olympics. Which of the following might preclude her clearance for gymnastics?
   a. Developmental disability
   b. Hypothyroidism
   c. Asthma
   d. Bipolar disorder

6. The preparticipation examination should be com-pleted at least 6 weeks before the start of the sports event or practice so that
   a. any identified problems can be rehabilitated.
   b. there is enough time to fill out the paperwork.
   c. orthopedic evaluation by a specialist can be completed.
   d. specialized neurologic evaluations can be completed.

7. A 17-year-old male patient has a history of head in-jury after a football injury. He returns for a prepar-ticipation examination for martial arts. Which of the following is true for this patient?
   a. Forty percent of high school athletes sustain a brain injury.
   b. He is ineligible for sports because of previous brain injury.
   c. He is only eligible for sports with low static demands.
   d. He has two to four times the probability of sustain-ing another head injury.

8. Which of the following is true regarding the prepar-ticipation examination?
   a. The only necessary component is a musculoskeletal examination.
   b. There is nothing legally binding about the provider's recommendation.
   c. Noncontact sports do not require a preparticipation examination.
   d. The only place to perform a preparticipation examination is in a clinic.

9. During the orthopedic component of the participa-tion examination, what is the purpose of identifying asymmetries of range of motion, strength, and muscle bulk?
   a. To center the examination on low-yield areas of importance
   b. To identify acute or old, poorly rehabilitated injuries
   c. To identify recommended types of activity limitation
   d. All of the above

10. Sudden cardiac death in athletes is a great concern. Which of the following precludes an athlete from participation in sports?
    a. Hypertension
    b. Carditis
    c. Heart murmur
    d. Dysrhythmia

11. You are evaluating a 19-year-old patient with Down syndrome for a preparticipation physical examina-tion. He is going to attend the Special Olympics and plans to play soccer. Which of the following would disqualify him for sports participation?
    a. Intellectual disability
    b. Type of sport he is playing
    c. Atlantoaxial instability
    d. Overweight

12. You are evaluating a patient after concussion for the ability to return to playing soccer. He is now doing noncontact training drills, but he is having some balance disturbance. Per the return to play protocol, you advise
a. 7 days of rest.
b. 5 days of rest and then return to play at the first step of the protocol.
c. 24 hours of rest and then return to play at the first step of the protocol.
d. 24 hours of rest and then return to sports specific exercise without head impact.

13. Which of the following conditions are reasons to deny a patient the ability to play sports?
a. Previous concussion
b. Heat-related illness
c. Fever
d. Hypertension

14. Harry is a 16-year-old patient who is returning for hypertension that is stage 2. This is defined as
a. blood pressure greater than the 99th percentile.
b. blood pressure greater than the 95th percentile.
c. blood pressure higher than 5mm Hg.
d. blood pressure greater than 110/80 mm Hg.

15. Which of the following are classified as limited contact sports?
a. Ultimate Frisbee and canoeing in white water
b. Bicycling and racquetball
c. Badminton and baseball
d. Lacrosse and diving

24 Putting it all Together

LEARNING OBJECTIVES

After studying Chapter 24 in the textbook and completing this section of the laboratory manual, students should be able to:
1. Discuss the process of completing the history and physical examination.
2. Describe patient reliability and factors that may affect the accuracy of the data collected.
3. Describe the general examination sequence.
4. Identify techniques useful for the evaluation of infants and young children.
5. Discuss the functional assessment.

TEXTBOOK REVIEW

Chapter 24: Putting it all Together (pp. 594–609)

CHAPTER OVERVIEW

This chapter focuses on the integration of previous chapters that included interviewing, building a history, and performing a physical examination. This chapter examines the physical examination sequence, discussing patient positioning and its relation to the specific examinations completed. Techniques for examining infants, children, pregnant women, older adults, and adult patients are compared. Finally, this chapter summarizes a functional assessment for an older adult.

TERMINOLOGY REVIEW

Activities of daily living (ADLs)—activities of daily living.

Basic activities of daily living—bathing, dressing, toileting, ambulation, and feeding.

Cultural barriers—pay attention to the possibility of cultural differences between you and the patient; approach the variety of life experience with candor and interested, compassionate inquiry (see page 595 in the textbook).

Emotional constraints, apparent and inapparent—patients who are psychotic, delirious, depressed, or in any way seriously emotionally affected may confuse you; emphasize mental status during the history when you suspect this.

Functional assessment—essential examination of every older adult whether this is one who is well or not coping well in the community environment.

Instrumental activities of daily living—housekeeping, grocery shopping, meal preparation, medication compliance, communication skills, and money management.

Language barriers—patients may speak a language different from yours; translation can be difficult in the best of circumstances; passing messages among three persons often results in changes in meaning that might have serious importance, and confusion may be the result; even using the same language may be a problem if the patient has a limited vocabulary, speaks English as a second language, or cannot read English very well.

Sensory deprivation—a partial or total loss of any of the senses (e.g., vision, hearing, touch, smell) is clearly constraining.

APPLICATION TO CLINICAL PRACTICE

Matching

Mr. Walker is a 62-year-old man requiring a routine physical examination. Listed below are some of the procedures that will be performed during the examination, as well as some of the equipment that will be needed. Match each examination procedure with type of equipment needed for the procedure. Some equipment will be used more than once; some procedures require more than one answer.

Examination Procedure	Equipment Needed
_____ 1. Red reflex	a. Eye chart (Snellen)
_____ 2. Lung sounds	b. Gloves
_____ 3. Jugular venous pulsations	c. Lubricant
_____ 4. Symmetry of muscle groups	d. Marking pen
_____ 5. Gag reflex	e. Measuring tape
_____ 6. Thyroid	f. Ophthalmoscope
_____ 7. Rectal and prostate examination	g. Otoscope
_____ 8. Tympanic membrane	h. Penlight
_____ 9. Visual acuity	i. Percussion hammer
_____ 10. Rinne and Weber tests	j. Stethoscope
_____ 11. Liver span	k. Tongue blade
_____ 12. Lymph nodes	l. Tuning fork
_____ 13. Heart murmurs	m. No equipment needed
_____ 14. Deep tendon reflex	
_____ 15. Romberg test	
_____ 16. Retinal examination	
_____ 17. Bowel sounds	
_____ 18. Tactile fremitus	

Concepts Application

Complete the following table by identifying the body systems examined in each of the examination areas listed in the left column. Select the appropriate body systems from the list provided below. You will use some systems more than once.

Auditory	Mouth and oropharynx
Breasts and axillae	Musculoskeletal
Cardiovascular	Neurologic
Gastrointestinal	Nose and paranasal
Integumentary	Respiratory
Lymphatic	Visual

Examination Area	Body Systems Examined
Upper extremities	
Anterior chest	
Abdomen	
Head and neck	

CRITICAL THINKING

1. A 61-year-old blind woman presents for a yearly physical examination. What type of modification, if any, should be made to individualize your examination approach or procedures for this individual?

2. A 43-year-old man presents for his 6-month physical examination. He has multiple health problems, including diabetes and coronary artery disease. From the onset of the examination, the patient is overbearing; he begins questioning your techniques and your abilities. He indicates that he is an important person in the community and knows many other people of importance. What things can you do to gain this individual's confidence and decrease his anxiety?

CONTENT REVIEW QUESTIONS

Multiple Choice

Circle the correct answer for each of the following questions.

1. When performing a physical examination, you should consider the examination to begin
   a. as soon as you meet the patient.
   b. after the vital signs are taken.
   c. after you explain to the patient everything you are going to do.
   d. after the patient has put on an examination gown.

2. The examiner may decide to omit various aspects of an examination. Which of the following is the best reason for this decision?
   a. The patient is feeling ill.
   b. The patient already knows what is wrong, and a diagnosis can be based on the history.
   c. Certain examination steps will provide data of limited value.
   d. Anxiety is observed by the examiner.

3. In what way can the patient's modesty be maintained while an examination is being conducted? The examiner should
   a. turn his or her back while the patient undresses.
   b. keep the patient covered as much as possible during the examination.
   c. avoid touching the patient during the examination except when absolutely necessary.
   d. not require the patient to disrobe for the examination.

4. Which examination approach is suggested for a 14-month-old baby? The baby should be
   a. completely undressed and lying down on an examination table.
   b. fully clothed and placed on the floor with toys; the examiner should conduct the examination while the child plays.
   c. completely undressed and held by the examiner.
   d. wearing only a diaper and sitting on his or her parent's lap.

5. Which examination technique is not generally included in the examination of a newborn infant?
   a. Percussion of the chest
   b. Palpation of the abdomen
   c. Auscultation of the lungs
   d. Inspection of the mouth and palate

6. Which of the following assists the examiner in determining the gestational age of a newborn infant?
   a. Measurement of the head circumference
   b. Percussion to determine liver size
   c. Inspection of hair distribution of the scalp
   d. Inspection of the sole of the foot

7. A patient complains of a sore throat. Which aspect of the examination could be eliminated?
   a. Vital signs
   b. Palpation of lymph nodes
   c. Deep tendon reflexes
   d. Auscultation of the heart and lungs

8. All of the following can be assessed initially during the general inspection *except*
   a. mobility.
   b. nutritional status.
   c. urinary function.
   d. skin color.

9. What technique will most likely facilitate the examination of a small frightened girl?
   a. Promise the child you won't hurt her.
   b. Tell the child a story in order to distract her.
   c. Use restraints to hold the child but tell her you are playing a game with her.
   d. Tell the child you will give her a toy or treat if she does not cry.

10. Which of the following is most relevant to the examination of an older adult?
    a. Functional assessment
    b. Physical measurements
    c. Developmental scoring
    d. Vital signs, including peripheral pulse examination

11. For a routine physical examination, all of the following equipment is necessary *except*
    a. penlight.
    b. measuring tape.
    c. examination gloves.
    d. monofilament.

12. Which of the following best describes when the collection of a history should be done?
    a. At the beginning of an examination to help identify problems
    b. At the end of the physical examination after problems are identified
    c. Before, during, and after the examination
    d. Only when relevant to the situation

13. Mr. Young is an 88-year-old man who comes to the office with his daughter for a follow-up. His daughter reports that he is not able to complete meal preparation, and she brings him meals daily. You document this as
    a. patient is unable to complete ADLs.
    b. patient is unable to complete basic ADLs.
    c. patient is unable to complete instrumental ADLs.
    d. patient requires assistance with meal preparation.

14. One way to adapt to the circumstance and use your clinical judgment is to
    a. expand on historical information or omit steps as needed.
    b. follow the system approach and do not deviate from the list.
    c. assess basic needs first and then more significant ones later.
    d. use close-ended questions to gather the significant findings.

15. The Ballard Gestational Age Score is completed within 36 hours of birth to
    a. determine if the menstrual-estimated age is correct.
    b. determine if the newborn is premature.
    c. determine an actual quantitative measure.
    d. combine objective and subjective observations.

Taking the Next Steps: Critical Thinking

LEARNING OBJECTIVES

After studying Chapter 25 in the textbook and completing this section of the laboratory manual, students should be able to:

1. Discuss the process of data analysis.
2. Describe barriers to critical thinking in reaching diagnostic conclusions.
3. Identify terms associated with data analysis and problem identification.
4. Discuss the role of additional testing in the clinical examination process.
5. Describe what is meant by a patient management plan and explain where it fits with critical thinking and clinical examination.

TEXTBOOK REVIEW

Chapter 25: Taking the Next Steps: Clinical Judgment (pp. 610–615)

CHAPTER OVERVIEW

This chapter examines the use of critical thinking and evidence-based practice as parts of the clinical decision-making process. Several barriers to critical thinking are categorized, including feelings, attitudes, and values of the clinician and patient. Bayes formula is evaluated in relation to critical thinking and clinical decision making. Finally, the reliability and validity of the clinical examination are discussed in relation to critical thinking.

TERMINOLOGY REVIEW

Bayes formula—the likelihood of a diagnosis being related to the findings depends on the probability of those findings being associated with that diagnosis.

Behavior change—a process involving progress through a series of stages.

Critical thinking—process by which the information gleaned from the history and physical examination is merged with clinical knowledge.

Evidence-based practice (EBP)—a system that incorporates the best available scientific evidence to clinical decision making in the care of the individual patient.

False negative—an observation made that suggests a condition is not present when it actually is present.

False positive—an observation made that suggests a condition is present when it is not.

Negative predictive value—the proportion of persons with an expected observation who ultimately prove not to have the expected condition (e.g., if 100 observations are made expecting a disease and 95 times that observation is not found and the condition proves not to have been the diagnosis, then the negative predictive value of the observation is 95%).

Occam's razor—a principle stating that all findings should be unified into one diagnosis; this is not always true.

Positive predictive value—the proportion of persons with an observation characteristic of a disease who actually have it (e.g., when an observation is made 100 times and on 95 of those occasions that observation proves to be consistent with the ultimate diagnosis, then the positive predictive value of the observation is 95%).

Sensitivity—the ability of an observation to identify correctly those who have a disease.

Specificity—the ability of an observation to identify correctly those who do not have the disease.

True negative—an expected observation that is not found when the disease characterized by that observation is not present.

True positive—an expected observation that is found when the disease characterized by that observation is present.

Concepts Application

Complete the following table by identifying the body systems that might be involved with each of the symptoms listed in the left column below. Choose body systems from the following list. All symptoms have more than one possible body system involvement, and body systems can be used more than once.

Auditory   Musculoskeletal
Cardiovascular   Neurologic
Gastrointestinal   Respiratory
Integumentary   Visual

Symptoms	Body Systems that Might Be Involved
Chest pain	
Headaches	
Abdominal pain	
Pain in the legs	

Matching

Match each concept or method with the best example of its application.

Concept or Method	Example of Application
_____ 1. Recognizing patterns	a. Sore throats are common problems.
_____ 2. Sampling the universe	b. If it looks like a cat, it must be a cat.
_____ 3. Using algorithms	c. Including everything precludes missing anything.
_____ 4. Guidelines to decision making	d. Rigidly defined thought process precludes error.

Matching

Match each concept with the scenario in which the term is applied. Use each concept only once.

Scenario	Concept
_____ 1. The examiner notes a positive Homans sign in the absence of thrombophlebitis.	a. Bayes formula
_____ 2. Based on observations, the examiner correctly concludes that a patient does not have renal disease.	b. False negative c. False positive
_____ 3. The patient does not demonstrate tenderness at the McBurney point and does not have appendicitis.	d. Negative predictive value
_____ 4. A numeric value is assigned, predicting the probability that a patient with negative findings does not have a given illness.	e. Positive predictive value
_____ 5. A diagnosis of hepatitis B infection is made based on the patient's symptoms and the population of IV drug abusers, of which he is part.	f. Sensitivity
_____ 6. The examiner correctly concludes that a patient has chronic hypoxia based on the patient's presentation.	g. Specificity
_____ 7. A patient with cholecystitis has a positive Murphy sign.	h. True positive
_____ 8. The examiner notes normal findings in a patient with prostate cancer.	i. True negative
_____ 9. With acute myocardial infarction, 90% of patients demonstrate diaphoresis.	

Concepts Application

Complete the following table by listing possible problems associated with the examination data provided.

Examination Data	Possible Problems
A 54-year-old woman with jaundice, abdominal pain, nausea, and weight loss. Has pain with abdominal palpation; positive bowel sounds. Liver slightly enlarged; admits to alcohol use.	
A 66-year-old man with a chief complaint of breathing difficulty. Has increased respiratory rate, low-grade fever, rales, productive cough; increased tactile fremitus bilaterally.	
A 13-week-old infant girl with fever, irritability, poor eating. Infant is dehydrated and has a temperature of 103.7° F; soft abdomen.	
A 19-year-old female college student with a chief complaint of pain when urinating. Describes frequency and urgency. Patient has temperature of 100.4° F; has constant pain in pelvic area; positive pain with fist percussion over left flank.	

Multiple Choice

Circle the correct answer for each of the following questions.

1. Unless a life-threatening situation exists, the best guide to determining the priority for the patient's condition should be based on
   a. intuition.
   b. probability and utility.
   c. the use of algorithms.
   d. the examiner's initial favorite hypothesis.

2. When determining a need for additional examination, testing, or procedures, the examiner knows that these should be done
   a. to obtain as much data as possible.
   b. to attempt to obtain data that might be associated with multiple problems.
   c. only when it is absolutely necessary.
   d. if they relate to the examiner's hypothesis.

3. After an examiner has identified and confirmed a problem, the next step is to
   a. assess the data collected.
   b. formulate a clinical opinion.
   c. conduct further assessment.
   d. determine the management plan.

4. The use of a computer could potentially be detrimental to the examiner because
   a. it may become a substitute for critical thinking.
   b. computer malfunction makes it unreliable.
   c. the computer is limited in the amount of data it can interpret.
   d. the level of skill needed to run a diagnostic computer program is beyond the computer skills of most examiners.

5. To identify problems based on clinical examination, the examiner should organize the data
   a. by dividing data into normal and abnormal findings.
   b. by body systems.
   c. by chief complaints.
   d. in the order the data were collected.

6. Each of the following could become a barrier to the critical thinking process, *except* for the examiner's
   a. feelings.
   b. attitudes.
   c. values.
   d. objectivity.

7. Which statement best characterizes a belief that supports a sound decision-making process?
   a. The underlying problem is always related to the chief complaint.
   b. Rare problems tend to have unusual presentations.
   c. Common problems occur commonly, and rare ones occur rarely.
   d. A diagnosis should be made quickly to enhance patient confidence.

8. Laboratory tests should be used to:
   a. confirm a presumed diagnosis.
   b. develop a list of potential problems.
   c. rule out all possible causes of symptoms and clinical findings.
   d. assist the examiner only when the data do not point to a specific problem.

9. Mr. David is a 62-year-old patient who has been diagnosed with alcohol addiction. After discussing his situation, he tells you that he is intending to take action regarding his alcohol use in the immediate future. Which stage of change is he in?
   a. Contemplation
   b. Action
   c. Preparation
   d. Precontemplation

10. EBP is defined as
    a. the best available scientific evidence to clinical decision making.
    b. translating decision making into patient care.
    c. a balance of treatment or lack of treatment.
    d. use of critical thinking to determine best diagnosis.

26 Recording Information

LEARNING OBJECTIVES

After studying Chapter 26 in the textbook and completing this section of the laboratory manual, students should be able to:
1. Describe reasons for maintaining clear and accurate records.
2. Discuss various components of the problem-oriented medical record set out in terminology review below.
3. Organize data in appropriate system sections of the history.
4. Delineate methods for documenting the location and description of findings.

TEXTBOOK REVIEW

Recording Information (pp. 616-631)

CHAPTER OVERVIEW

This chapter examines the components of recording information for the medical record so that you and your colleagues can care for the patient, identifying health problems, making diagnoses and judgments of diagnostic testing needed, planning appropriate care, and monitoring the patient's response to treatment. The proper organization of the health history and physical examination findings in the appropriate section of the medical record is reviewed. Also discussed is the importance of accurate documentation of the findings in a medical record. Finally, methods for documenting the location and description of findings are delineated.

TERMINOLOGY REVIEW

Chief concern—a brief description of the patient's main reason for seeking care, stated verbatim in quotation marks.
Comprehensive health history and physical examination—record that must include all data collected, both positive and negative, that contribute to the examiner's assessment.
Episodic illness visit—scenario in which a patient seeks care for an acute problem, which is usually rapidly resolved.
Family history—includes a pedigree with at least three generations; it also includes major health or genetic disorders.
History of present illness—a detailed description of all symptoms may be related to the chief concern; describes the concern for problem chronologically, dating events and symptoms.
OLDCARTS mnemonic—onset, location, duration, character, aggravating factors, relieving factors, temporal factors, and severity of symptoms.
Past medical history—includes general health over the patient's lifetime as well as disabilities and functional limitations as the patient perceives them.
Personal and social history—this area includes cultural background, birthplace, education, family, marital status, general life satisfaction, hobbies, sources of stress, and religious practices.
Plan—a list of interventions divided into three categories—diagnosis, treatment, and patient education—based on each problem in the problem list.
Problem list—a running log of problem number, date of onset, description of problem, and date the problem was resolved.
Problem-oriented medical record (POMR)—a format for recording health history and physical examination findings by documenting the problem assessment process.
Progress notes—part of the medical record in which health history and physical examination findings are documented in a variety of formats.

Concepts Application 1

Fill in the blanks in the following statements, selecting appropriate terms from the list below.

Subjective	Chief concern
SOAP	Objective
Illustration	Health history
POMR	Incremental grading
	Physical examination

1. _____ data are collected during the history and are based on patient reports.

2. A brief description of the patient's main reason for seeking health care is referred to as the _____ .

3. _____ A format used to document health history notes especially for care beyond the initial evaluation.

4. The use of stick people to document findings is an example of using a(n) _____ .

5. _____ data are collected while conducting the physical examination.

6. _____ This is the use of recorded numbers to represent findings by variable degrees.

7. This _____ is a widely accepted medical record format consisting of six components.

8. This _____ is the part of the record where information from a patient interview is recorded.

9. Clinical findings are recorded during the _____ .

Concepts Application 2

Develop a problem list for Mrs. Olivas based on the following information.

Mrs. Olivas comes to the clinic complaining of back pain. She indicates this pain started in June 1998 while she was moving some rocks in her garden. Other pertinent aspects of her history include insulin-dependent diabetes mellitus since 1977, which she says she has never really had under control, and cholecystitis, for which she had a cholecystectomy in May 1997. Mrs. Olivas has a family history of atherosclerotic heart disease and chronic renal failure.

Problem #	Onset	Problem	Date Resolved
1.	June 1998	Low back pain	Ongoing
2.			
3.			
4.			
5.			

Case Study

Jean is a 37-year-old woman who has been interviewed for a health history. Her family history is provided in the following paragraph. Below the paragraph, draw a genogram for Jean's family history using the information provided.

Jean is married. Her husband is 43 years old. They have a 12-year-old son, an 11-year-old daughter, and a 10-year-old son, all in good health. Jean has a 42-year-old brother and three sisters, 40, 36, and 32 years of age. All of her siblings are in good health. Both of Jean's parents are alive. Her 70-year-old father has mild emphysema and is an only child. Her mother is 66 years old and has hypertension. Jean's mother has three siblings; the oldest (Jean's uncle) is 74 years old and has glaucoma. Another brother is 72 years old and is in good health. A sister is 69 years old and has osteoarthritis. All of Jean's grandparents are deceased. Her paternal grandfather died at the age of 89 years of prostate cancer. Her paternal grandmother died of congestive heart failure at the age of 91 years. Jean's maternal grandfather died at the age of 86 years of prostate cancer, and her maternal grandmother died at 96 years of "old age."

CRITICAL THINKING

1. The onset of a "new" symptom should be thoroughly documented. Describe what the mnemonic device "OLDCARTS" refers to regarding documentation of a symptom.

   O:

   L:

   D:

   C:

   A:

   R:

   T:

   S:

2. While examining a patient, you note a mass. What characteristics should be described when documenting any organ, mass, or lesion?

Multiple Choice

Circle the correct answer for each of the following questions.

1. Which of the following examples illustrates a vague or nondescriptive term?
   a. "Skin color is normal."
   b. "Skin turgor is elastic."
   c. "Skin is thin and smooth."
   d. "Skin is warm and dry."

2. How are "normal findings" best documented?
   a. Write "normal" or "within normal limits" on the documentation form.
   b. Write "NA" (not applicable) on the documentation sheet.
   c. Because documentation focuses on abnormal findings, do not write anything for normal findings.
   d. Document what was actually assessed in specific terms.

3. One way that a health history for an infant differs from that of an adult is the inclusion of
   a. nutritional history.
   b. chief concern.
   c. prenatal information.
   d. personal social information.

4. If a mistake is made in the patient record, it is suggested that a line be drawn through the mistake so that it is still legible. The basis for this action is related to the fact that
   a. no errors are allowed.
   b. the chart is a legal document.
   c. a pen is messy when used to obliterate writing.
   d. others may want to read what your first impressions were.

5. Which of the following statements is true regarding use of abbreviations?
   a. Use of any abbreviations is fine as long as you can interpret them.
   b. Abbreviations should be used as much as possible to reduce time and space needed for documentation.
   c. Abbreviations should be avoided because they are not considered acceptable.
   d. Use only universally accepted abbreviations for documentation.

6. The examiner can substantially reduce the possibility of legal problems by
   a. maintaining clear medical records.
   b. using the SOAP format to document all entries.
   c. using a POMR.
   d. drawing genograms in the patient record.

7. Which of the following information belongs in a family history?
   a. Chronic illness
   b. Current problems
   c. Hereditary diseases
   d. Personal data

8. A drawing in the medical record may be used to document
   a. pulse amplitude.
   b. location of lesions.
   c. location of a mass.
   d. all of the above.

9. You are taking a health history on your patient. When you are asking about problems in other body systems, your patient reports constipation over the past 5 or 6 months. This would be documented in
   a. chief complaint.
   b. past medical history.
   c. review of systems.
   d. assessment.

10. Your patient presents to the office with a chief complaint of shoulder pain that he reports as stabbing. In using the mnemonic OLDCARTS, this is noted as
    a. character.
    b. duration.
    c. location.
    d. onset.

Emergency or Life-Threatening Situations

LEARNING OBJECTIVES

After studying Chapter 27 in the textbook and completing this section of the laboratory manual, students should be able to:
1. Compare and contrast primary and secondary assessment.
2. Describe findings considered significant in the secondary assessment.
3. Describe how pediatric emergency assessment differs from adult emergency assessment.
4. Identify pediatric findings considered to be of concern or ominous.
5. Discuss the impact of advance directives on providing immediate care.

TEXTBOOK REVIEW

Chapter 27: Emergency or Life-Threatening Situations (pp. 632-644)

CHAPTER OVERVIEW

This chapter examines emergency situations and the primary and secondary assessments necessary to care for these specialized patients. This assessment must take seconds, not minutes. The ABCs of a primary assessment are analyzed, as are the components of a thorough secondary assessment. In addition, this chapter illustrates the assessment components and techniques for a variety of emergency situations, such as trauma and burns. Finally, the chapter reviews the legal considerations in caring for patients in emergency situations.

TERMINOLOGY REVIEW

ABCs—airway, breathing, circulation.
Advance directive—a formal statement of desired medical care in the event of catastrophic injury or illness.
Blunt trauma—injury that does not penetrate the skin.
Durable power of attorney—a provision for another person to make health care decisions in the event that the patient's cognition is lost.
Hypoxemia—severely reduced blood oxygen levels in major organs, resulting from respiratory distress, poor tissue perfusion, or ventilatory failure.
Increased intracranial pressure—a condition in which an increase in the volume of brain tissue, blood, or cerebrospinal fluid within the closed space of the skull results in elevated pressure.
Penetrating trauma—injury that penetrates the patient's skin.
Primary assessment—rapid evaluation of the patient's physiologic status (the ABCs).
Pulmonary embolism—migration of a blood clot from the deep veins of the legs or pelvis to the lung vasculature.
Secondary assessment—more detailed head-to-toe examination to identify problems.
Shock state—abnormality of the circulatory system that results in inadequate organ perfusion and tissue oxygenation; common causes include hemorrhage associated with injury.
Status asthmaticus—acute severe asthma exacerbation that does not respond to usual treatment.
Status epilepticus—a prolonged seizure (or a series of seizures) that occurs without recovery of consciousness.
Upper airway obstruction—compromise of the airway space resulting in impaired respiratory exchange.
Ventilatory failure—compromised exhalation of carbon dioxide caused by alveolar hypoventilation.

APPLICATION TO CLINICAL PRACTICE

Concepts Application

Indicate whether the action described would be part of a primary or secondary assessment in a patient with a life-threatening condition.

1. _____ Removing clothing from a patient with an abdominal gunshot wound

2. _____ Performing a Glasgow Coma Scale assessment

3. _____ Taking a history of injury

4. _____ Stabilizing the cervical spine

5. _____ Auscultating the heart

6. _____ Taking vital signs

7. _____ Managing a large, pulsating, bleeding wound

8. _____ Assessing for presence of breathing

9. _____ Assessing the abdomen for internal bleeding

10. _____ Conducting diagnostic tests

11. _____ Assessing peripheral pulses

Case Study

Mark O'Neil is a 19-year-old man rushed to the emergency department by his roommate.

PRIMARY ASSESSMENT

Upon arrival, Mark is extremely anxious and has profound dyspnea. He states, "Please help me. I can't breathe enough air—something is wrong with me! My chest hurts all over, and I can't breathe!" The examiner notes a large, muscular, healthy-appearing man in acute respiratory distress. Nasal flaring is noted with cyanosis around the lips. Overall impression is that of hypoxia.

1. Based on this information, list your primary assessment findings:
   A:

   B:

   C:

2. What type of treatment should be initiated immediately during the primary assessment?

3. What is the first thing that should be assessed at the onset of the secondary assessment?

SECONDARY ASSESSMENT: SUBJECTIVE DATA

Mark's roommate tells you that Mark is very athletic and very healthy. "He plays college football and had surgery on his knee 2 weeks ago because of an injury this past season. This evening he was fine—we were watching TV. Then when he got up to go into the kitchen, he called for help and told me to get him to the hospital now! All that happened about 20 minutes ago." The roommate says that Mark does not use any drugs. He adds, "He drinks beer and stuff, but nothing tonight."

SECONDARY ASSESSMENT: OBJECTIVE DATA

Vital signs: Pulse 142. Respiratory rate 40. Blood pressure 138/84. Temperature 99.1°F.

Skin color: Generally pale with cyanosis around lips and in nail beds.

Head/neck: Pupils reactive to light. Oral cavity WNL.

Chest: Breath sounds auscultated in all lung fields. Has productive cough with bloody sputum. Heart sounds WNL.

Abdomen: Bowel sounds present. No pain; soft, nondistended.

Extremities: Pulses palpable in all extremities; no swelling.

Neurologic: Awake but not following all commands; extremely anxious.

Arterial blood gas: pH 7.31; O_2 63; PCO_2 69 (respiratory acidosis).

4. What data deviate from normal?

5. What additional secondary assessment would you plan to conduct?

6. Based on the information presented, what problems do you think this patient might be experiencing?

Matching

Match each clinical sign to the condition(s) with which it is likely to be associated. Answers may be used more than once; some conditions have more than one answer.

Condition	Clinical Sign
_____ 1. Ectopic pregnancy	a. Battle sign
_____ 2. Pneumothorax	b. Cullen sign
_____ 3. Basilar skull fracture	c. Grey-Turner sign
_____ 4. Retroperitoneal hematoma	d. Hamman sign
_____ 5. Facial fracture	e. Kehr sign
_____ 6. Blunt injury to abdomen	f. Raccoon eyes

CRITICAL THINKING

1. Mrs. Martin and her 3-year-old daughter, Amanda, are brought to the hospital for emergency care after being burned in a house fire.
   a. In addition to the burns, what types of problems should the examiner rule out on both of these patients?

   b. What anatomic differences between Amanda and her mother will affect how they are examined?

CONTENT REVIEW QUESTIONS

Multiple Choice
Circle the correct answer for each of the following questions.

1. Approximately how long should an examiner take to conduct a primary assessment of a stable patient?
   a. 30 seconds
   b. 60 seconds
   c. 2 minutes
   d. 5 minutes

2. After the initial primary assessment is conducted, how often should it be repeated?
   a. Every 30 seconds
   b. Every 2 minutes
   c. Every 5 minutes
   d. Every time the patient's condition changes

3. Which finding is consistent with abdominal hemorrhage?
   a. Increased bowel sounds
   b. Distention and pain
   c. Hyperresonance with percussion
   d. Auscultation of mesentery artery

4. Which of the following findings suggests a serious problem in a 3-year-old child who has fallen from a tree?
   a. Respiratory rate of 38 breaths/min
   b. Pulse rate of 150 beats/min
   c. Lethargy
   d. Crying

5. Mike complains of severe rib pain. His coworkers state that he was hurt on the job when a large pipe struck him across the chest. Given this history, which type of problem should be considered during the secondary assessment?
   a. Flail chest
   b. Rebound tenderness
   c. Pulmonary embolus
   d. Pupillary constriction

6. A patient who was involved in a motor vehicle accident presents with a suspected neck injury. Which of the following actions by the examiner is clearly *not* appropriate?
   a. Assessing peripheral pulses
   b. Providing airway support
   c. Logrolling the patient to assess his back
   d. Hyperextending the neck to establish an airway

7. With which of the following clinical problems would crepitation be an expected finding?
   a. Myocardial infarction
   b. Cardiovascular accident
   c. Blunt abdominal trauma
   d. Pneumothorax

8. During the primary assessment, the examiner asks the patient, "Can you tell me who you are?" This question assesses
   a. airway and orientation.
   b. exposure and circulation.
   c. breathing and circulation.
   d. disability and exposure.

9. Which of the following findings suggests poor peripheral perfusion?
   a. Rapid heart rate
   b. Dorsalis pedis pulse with 3+ amplitude
   c. Capillary refill time longer than 2 seconds
   d. Radial pulse palpable

10. A child is struck by a car while riding his bike. Upon arrival at the hospital, the child is not breathing. Which of the following best describes the appropriate actions of an examiner?
    a. Conduct a primary and secondary assessment before deciding what care to provide.
    b. Conduct a primary assessment; before starting a secondary assessment, support breathing.
    c. Stop the primary assessment as soon as the apnea is recognized in order to perform interventions to stabilize the breathing.
    d. Appropriate action depends on the degree of cyanosis observed by the examiner.

11. A patient displays the Cushing triad (a drop in pulse rate, rise in blood pressure, and widened pulse pressure). With which type of life-threatening condition are such clinical findings associated?
    a. Myocardial infarction
    b. Ruptured cerebral aneurysm
    c. Status asthmaticus
    d. Status epilepticus

12. An examiner suspects that a patient has a cervical spine injury. The examiner can rule out this possibility by
    a. examining peripheral motor and sensation.
    b. assessing level of consciousness.
    c. assessing for pain and deformity.
    d. acquiring radiographic films of all cervical vertebrae.

13. During primary assessment, the examiner notes dampness inside a trauma victim's dark-colored coat. Which of the following possible causes for the dampness would be most important for the examiner to determine?
    a. Severe sweating
    b. Urine
    c. IV fluids
    d. Blood

14. A patient presents with a complaint of sudden flashes of light in the field of vision. What other symptom commonly accompanies this primary symptom?
    a. Severe nausea and vomiting
    b. Partial loss of vision
    c. Severe pain to the eye
    d. Intense dizziness

15. A man is shot and critically wounded during a domestic dispute. From a legal standpoint, the health care providers must
    a. obtain written consent from the patient before providing care.
    b. call the police before providing care.
    c. save all items obtained from the patient for law enforcement personnel.
    d. determine whether the man has advance directives before providing care.

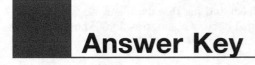

Answer Key

CHAPTER 1

Application to Clinical Practice

Case Study

1. The chief complaint is fatigue.

2. Questions to ask:
   When did the fatigue start?
   What does it feel like?
   How often does it occur?
   What factors have made it improve or get worse?
   How severe is the fatigue?

3. Systems to include in the ROS:
   General
   Skin
   Chest
   Cardiovascular
   Hematologic
   Diet
   Endocrine

Concepts Application

Patient Behavior	Examiner Behavior to Decrease Tension
Seduction	Do not respond to seductive behavior. Be courteous, calm, firm, and direct from the start; send the message that the relationship is, and will remain, professional.
Depression	Do not neglect it. Allow the interview to continue but come back with gentle questioning to indicate you think there may be more to the story than what has been discussed.
Anxiety	Avoid overload of information. Pace the conversation with a calm demeanor; avoid allowing the anxiety to become contagious.
Excessive flattery	Be aware that this is possibly a manipulation on the part of the patient; it is easy to be taken in by such manipulations.
Financial concerns	Be aware that the patient may be concerned about the cost of health care; be prepared to talk about it with the patient.
Silence	Be patient. Allow a moment of silence. Silence allows the patient a moment of reflection.

Critical Thinking

Case Study 1

1. O (onset)—started 2 weeks ago
   L (location)—outside edge of the heel of the left foot
   D (duration)—lasts 2 to 3 hours in the morning
   C (characteristic)—burning pain
   A (aggravating factors)—upon awakening in the morning and walking barefoot
   R (relieving factors)—ice and Tylenol one to two times per day.
   T (timing)—2 to 3 hours every day
   S (severity)—severe pain

Case Study 2

1. Components of a health history present in the case study:
   CC
   HPI
   ROS
   PMH
   SH

2. The FH should have been added to the health history.

3. Components that are only partially complete:
   ROS—additional head and neck and reproductive questions
   SH—living situation questions

Content Review Questions

Multiple Choice

1. c
2. c
3. b
4. c
5. d
6. a
7. b
8. b
9. a
10. c
11. c
12. a
13. c
14. c
15. b
16. d
17. d
18. d
19. a
20. b

CHAPTER 2

Application to Clinical Practice

Case Study

1. What do you call your problem?
   What do you think caused your problem?
   Why do you think it started when it did?
   What does your sickness do to you?
   How does it work?
   How bad is your sickness?
   How long do you think it will last?
   What should be done to get rid of it?
   Why did you come to me for treatment?
   What benefit will you get from treatment?
   What are the most important problems your sickness has caused for you?
   What worries you and frightens you the most about your sickness?
   Who else or what else might help you get better?
   Has anyone else helped you with this problem?

2. "People have told me that there are ways of treating sickness that doctors and nurses don't know about."
   "Do you know any of them? What are they?"
   "Do they work?"
   "Have you ever tried them?"
   "Do you use them?"
   "Are they helpful?"

3. Cereal grains and chili peppers

Concepts Application

1. Possible response of patient who is present oriented: "Why should I watch my diet? I only live for today; you never know what could happen tomorrow."
2. Possible response of patient who is future oriented: "I will make a plan to lose 8 pounds per month, create menu plans, and sign up at the gym because I want to live a long, happy life. I can overcome this."

Critical Thinking

Case Study 1

1. Hispanics have a collateral relational orientation in which the group's goals dominate over the individual's goals.
2. "Cold" foods include cod fish and fresh vegetables; "cold" medicines and herbs the patient might have tried include orange flower water and soda.

Case Study 2

1. *Health belief and practices:* What does illness mean to you? How do you perceive your health? What do you currently do to treat your illness and to help you stay healthy?
2. *Religious and ritual influences:* Do you have any special religious practices or beliefs? Are there any special practices you follow or beliefs you have about illness or dying?
3. *Dietary practices:* What does your family eat? Who prepares the food? How is the food prepared?
4. *Family relationships:* What are the roles of your family members? Who is responsible for child rearing?

Self Reflection: If you are unsure of your responses, please review the components of a cultural response on page 25 of your textbook.

Content Review Questions

Multiple Choice

1. b
2. d
3. c
4. d
5. a
6. b

7. b
8. c
9. a
10. c
11. b
12. d
13. d
14. a

CHAPTER 3

Application to Clinical Practice

Concepts Application 1

Description	Examination Technique or Equipment
Gathering information through touch	Palpation
Grid used to assess for macular degeneration	Amsler
The fifth vital sign	Pain
Source of light with a narrow beam	Transilluminator
Used to test deep tendon reflexes	Percussion hammer
Used to visualize turbinates	Nasal speculum
Assesses near vision	Rosenbaum or Jaeger chart
Measures skinfold thickness	Lange or Harpenden calipers
Larger field of view in eye examination	Pan-optic ophthalmoscope

Concepts Application 2

Area Percussed	Percussion Tone Expected
Stomach	Tympanic
Sternum	Flat
Lung of patient with emphysema	Hyperresonant
Liver	Dull
Lung of patient with pneumonia	Dull
Lung of normal patient	Resonant
Abdomen with large tumor	Dull

Critical Thinking

1. Place Mrs. Johnson in a separate room. Wear gloves with the examination. Properly dispose of any disposable items that come into contact with the patient. Disinfect the room and all nondisposable articles after the patient leaves.

2. a. Use plain soap for routine handwashing.
   b. Use an antimicrobial soap in an outbreak situation or when a specific infection is known.

3. a. Ask Mr. Helms to describe in what way his feet do not "feel right." Ask for more specific symptoms such as pain, numbness, or loss of movement. Complete a symptom analysis using the mnemonic OLDCARTS.
   b. The examiner should assess for the loss of protective sensation in the feet. A monofilament will help identify a patient with decreased sensation and increased risk for injury.

Content Review Questions

Multiple Choice

1. c
2. b
3. d
4. b
5. b
6. a
7. a
8. a
9. d
10. c
11. a
12. c
13. b
14. a
15. c
16. b
17. d
18. c
19. a
20. c
21. d
22. d
23. a
24. a
25. c
26. a
27. d
28. d

CHAPTER 4

Application to Clinical Practice

Case Study

1. *Onset:* Date of onset, duration, cyclic nature, variability, related to injury or exposure to illness
2. *Associated symptoms:* Sweating, chills, irritability, nausea, vomiting, fatigue
3. *Medications:* Acetaminophen or nonsteroidal antiinflammatory drugs

Case Study 2

Diagnosis	Pain Findings
General pain	Vital sign changes, pallor, diaphoresis, dry mouth, facial mask of pain, irritability
Carpal tunnel syndrome	
Gastroesophageal reflux disease	Burning, shocklike pain
Osteoarthritis	Cramping, guarding over abdomen
	Tender, deep, and aching pain

Critical Thinking

Case Study 1

1. Stiffness of blood vessels and increased vascular resistance
2. Because of increased vagal tone

Case Study 2

1. Guarding of the abdomen, change in vital signs, facial distortions, dry mouth, pupil dilation
2. Visceral or colic pain

Content Review Questions

Multiple Choice

1. a
2. d
3. b
4. c
5. a
6. d
7. b
8. b
9. a
10. d
11. a
12. a
13. c
14. c
15. a
16. a
17. b
18. a
19. b
20. c

172

Answer Key

CHAPTER 5

Application to Clinical Practice

Matching

1. d
2. b
3. f
4. a
5. c
6. e

Concepts Application

1. *Attention:* Recite a list of numbers slowly and have the patient repeat them in the correct order. The patient should be able to repeat the series of numbers correctly.
2. *Memory:* Give the patient a list of items to remember and have the list repeated back after a 5-minute interval. The patient should be able to recall the items correctly.
3. *Judgment:* Ask the patient hypothetical questions involving situations in which decisions must be made, such as finding money on the sidewalk or seeing a car on fire. The patient should be able to evaluate a situation and describe an appropriate action to take in the circumstances.
4. *Abstract reasoning:* Recite a common proverb to the patient and request an explanation of its meaning. The patient should be able to give appropriate interpretations within his cultural frame of reference.
5. *Thought processes and content:* Observe the patient's pattern of thought during the interview and examination process. The patient should be logical, coherent, and goal oriented.

Case Study

1. Data deviating from normal: The patient recently lost her spouse. Son says his mother has "gone downhill." Son indicates patient is no longer keeping her house clean or cooking appropriate meals. Son reports significant change in patient's personal hygiene habits. Son reports that patient becomes angry when he talks about other living options. Patient states, "You think I am helpless and want to lock me away." Patient is 78-year-old woman who sits quietly during conversation. Overall hygiene is clean, but her hair is matted, and her clothes are wrinkled and do not match. Overall affect is very dull; she makes no eye contact with her son or the examiner.
2. The examiner should ask questions related to cognitive abilities and emotional stability.
3. The examiner should conduct a physical examination that will provide clues to her cognitive abilities as well as her emotional stability.
4. The patient may have depression.

Critical Thinking

1. **Depression** is associated with grief, a stressful life event, a reaction to medical or neurologic diseases, or a change in lifestyle. It may occur suddenly or slowly and is characterized by impaired concentration, reduced attention span, indecisiveness, slower thought processes, and impaired short- and long-term memory. The patient often feels sad, hopeless, and worthless and has a loss of interest or pleasure, but there are no delusions or hallucinations. Insomnia or excessive sleeping, fatigue, restlessness, anxiety, and increased or decreased appetite may also occur. Depression can be treated, and it can recur.

   Delirium may be associated with infections, medications, electrolyte and metabolic disorders, major organ failure, brain insults, and acute alcohol withdrawal; it lasts for hours or days. It is characterized by a sudden onset, altered consciousness; impaired memory, attentiveness, and consciousness; rapid mood swings; rambling and illogical or incoherent speech; and increased or decreased activity. Misperceptions, illusions, hallucinations, and delusions are common. Delirium may be reversible.

   Dementia, associated with a structural disease of the brain, is characterized by a slow, persistent, and progressive course that cannot be reversed. Initially, the patient has minimal cognitive impairment, but as the disorder progresses, abstract thinking, judgment, memory, thought patterns, and calculations become impaired. Delusions may be present, but misperceptions and hallucinations are usually absent. Speech may become rambling and incoherent as the patient struggles to find words. Behavior is usually unchanged.

2. *Personality*: Although personality does not typically change, existing personality traits may become exaggerated.

   Intellectual function: Typically, intellectual function does not deteriorate before 70 years of age unless a disease process or medications affect it. Some individuals have problems understanding new concepts by 80 years of age.

   Problem-solving skills: There is a deterioration of problem-solving skills with aging, but it is thought that this may be a result of disuse.

   Memory: Short-term, or recent, memory typically deteriorates before distant memory.

Content Review Questions

Multiple Choice

1. d
2. c
3. b
4. a
5. c
6. b
7. c
8. a
9. b
10. c

CHAPTER 6

Critical Thinking

1. a. *Growth hormone:* Secreted by the pituitary gland
   b. *Growth hormone–releasing hormone (GHRH):* Stimulates the pituitary to release growth hormone
   c. *Somatostatin:* Inhibits secretion of both GHRH and thyroid-stimulating hormone
   d. *Insulin-like growth factor (IGF-I):* In conjunction with growth hormone, stimulates muscle and skeletal growth
2. a. *Sex steroids (androgens):* Stimulate increased secretion of the growth hormone, which mediates the increase in IGF-I
   b. *Testosterone:* Enhances muscular development and sexual maturation; promotes bone maturation and epiphyseal closure
   c. *Estrogen:* Stimulates development of secondary sex characteristics and skeletal maturation
3. Leptin has a key role in regulating body fat mass, and its concentration is thought to be a trigger for puberty by informing the central nervous system that adequate nutritional status and body fat mass are present to support pubertal changes and growth.

Matching

1. f
2. c
3. e
4. d
5. b
6. a

Content Review Questions

Multiple Choice

1. d
2. c
3. b
4. c
5. b
6. a
7. c
8. c
9. d
10. a
11. c
12. a

CHAPTER 7

Application to Clinical Practice

Case Study 1

1. Note: The formula necessary to complete this activity is from Table 7-1 in the textbook.
   15-year-old young man weighing 110 pounds: $(17.5 \times 110) + 651 = 2576$ kcal/day
   25-year-old woman weighing 142 pounds: $(14.7 \times 142) + 496 = 2583$ kcal/day
   32-year-old woman weighing 200 pounds: $(8.7 \times 200) + 829 = 2569$ kcal/day
   62-year old man weighing 168 pounds: $(13.5 \times 168) + 487 = 2755$ kcal/day

Case Study 2

1. Desirable body weight: 5 ft, 9 in $= 106 + (6 \times 9) = 160$ lb
2. Percentage of desirable body weight: $142/160 \times 100 = 88.75\%$
3. Percentage of usual body weight: $142/172 \times 100 = 82.56\%$
4. Percentage of weight change: $172 - 142/172 \times 100 = 17.44\%$
5. Current BMI = 21.08
6. Previous BMI = 25.55
7. 10th percentile
8. Based on all the calculations, Jack has had a significant loss in weight. A change of 17% body weight in a 9-month period of time is of great concern.

Matching

1. e
2. c
3. a
4. b
5. f
6. d

Critical Thinking

1. a. Carbohydrates are the main source of energy for humans. Carbohydrates are found mostly in plants and milk. Moderate amounts must be ingested frequently to meet the energy demands of the body.
   b. Protein is essential to life. Proteins are present in all animal and plant products. Twenty different amino acids combine in different ways to form proteins. Major functions of proteins include building and maintaining tissues; regulating internal water and acid–base balance; and acting as a precursor for enzymes, antibodies, and hormones.
   c. Fats are present in animal and certain plant products. Fat is necessary as the main source of linoleic acid and is essential for normal growth and development. Functions include synthesis and regulation of certain hormones, tissues, nerve impulse transmission, memory storage, and energy metabolism.
2. Vitamins, minerals, and electrolytes are essential for growth and development and for metabolic processes; they are not used for energy. These micronutrients must be taken in either by food or supplements.
3. The following micronutrients are synthesized by the body:
   Vitamin K and biotin, which are produced by intestinal microorganisms
   Vitamin D, which is synthesized from cholesterol
   Niacin, which is synthesized from tryptophan

174

Answer Key

Content Review Questions

Multiple Choice

1. c
2. c
3. a
4. b
5. a
6. b
7. b
8. d

9. c
10. b
11. c
12. d
13. a
14. b
15. c
16. b
17. d
18. d

CHAPTER 8

Application to Clinical Practice

Anatomy Review

a. Cuticle
b. Nail plate
c. Perionychium
d. Lunula
e. Eponychium

Concepts Application

Type of Lesion	Examples
1. Excoriation	Abrasion, scratch, scabies
2. Fissure	Athlete's foot, cracks at corner of mouth
3. Erosion	Varicella or variola after rupture
4. Ulcer	Decubitus ulcers, stasis ulcers

Matching 1

1. c
2. h
3. e
4. g
5. d
6. i
7. a
8. f
9. b

Matching 2

1. d
2. b
3. c
4. a

Matching 3

1. a
2. b
3. a
4. a
5. b
6. c
7. a
8. c

Case Study

1. All data described are considered normal for the age of the patient, with the exception of the ulcerations on the lower extremities. This could be caused by a number of factors, but it is definitely not within normal limits for any age.
2. Ask when he first noticed the lesions, how often he has had the lesions, and what seems to help them get better. Ask if he has any pain in his legs associated with activity.
3. Assess circulation to the feet. An ulcerated open wound that does not heal most likely indicates insufficient perfusion of blood leading to tissue anoxia. It is possible that a Doppler study may be needed to assess pulses, or vascular studies may need to be considered.
4. The most common reason for this problem is insufficient perfusion. This may be the result of underlying vascular disease or heart disease; it may also be associated with diabetes.

Critical Thinking

1. Explain the following ABCD early signs of melanoma to Mr. Mason:
   A = Asymmetry. Melanoma lesions are asymmetrical in shape and appearance.
   B = Border. Melanoma lesions have irregular, indistinct, and sometimes notched borders.
   C = Color. Melanoma lesions tend to have uneven and variegated color. Lesions may vary from brown to pink to purple or have a mixed pigmentation.
   D = Diameter. Melanoma lesions are usually greater than 6 cm (2 inches) in diameter.

2. The examiner should note the following: location (where the lesion is found), distribution (isolated lesions or confluent), color, size, pattern (clustered, linear), shape, elevation (flat, raised), and characteristics (hard, soft, crusty, fluid-filled, solid, draining).

Content Review Questions

Multiple Choice

1. a
2. c
3. a
4. b
5. d
6. c
7. c
8. d
9. b
10. a
11. a
12. a
13. a
14. b
15. c
16. a
17. d
18. b
19. b
20. d

CHAPTER 9

Application to Clinical Practice

Anatomy Review

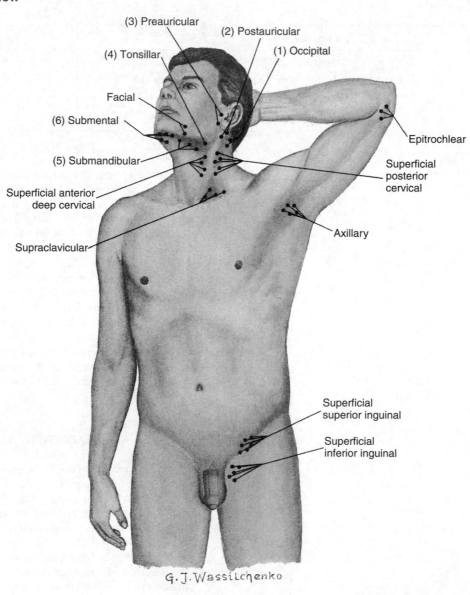

(3) Preauricular
(2) Postauricular
(4) Tonsillar
(1) Occipital
Facial
(6) Submental
Epitrochlear
(5) Submandibular
Superficial posterior cervical
Superficial anterior deep cervical
Supraclavicular
Axillary
Superficial superior inguinal
Superficial inferior inguinal

G.J. Wassilchenko

Matching

1. i
2. c
3. h
4. a
5. d
6. g
7. f
8. b
9. e

Case Study

1. Data deviating from normal: Fatigue and weakness, enlarged lymph nodes
2. Ask whether there is tenderness to the lymph nodes. Ask whether the patient has been ill recently. Ask whether he has had recent weight loss, has been eating properly, and has been getting adequate sleep.
3. Assess lymph nodes in neck, axilla, arm, and groin. Compare palpable lymph nodes for symmetry. Note the size, consistency, mobility, borders, and tenderness of lymph nodes.
4. Enlarged lymph nodes could be the result of a recent viral infection or a more serious problem such as a lymphoma or malignancy.

Critical Thinking

1. Compared with that of an adult, the lymph system of an infant or small child is proportionally much larger (the thymus, in particular, is quite large). Lymph nodes are normally readily palpable. After puberty, the lymph nodes become small and much less pronounced. The thymus shrinks to a point where it is not assessed. By the time an adult reaches late adult years, the lymph nodes become very small and have limited function. The nodes become fibrotic and fatty and become impaired in their ability to resist infection.

Content Review Questions

Multiple Choice

1. a
2. d
3. b
4. c
5. b
6. b
7. c
8. c
9. a
10. d
11. c

12. d
13. b
14. c
15. a
16. a
17. c
18. d

CHAPTER 10

Application to Clinical Practice

Matching

1. d
2. c
3. a
4. e
5. b

Anatomy Review

a. Hyoid bone
b. External carotid artery
c. Thyroid cartilage
d. Internal jugular vein
e. Common carotid artery
f. Thyroid gland
g. Right subclavian artery
h. Right subclavian vein
i. Brachiocephalic artery and vein
j. Internal carotid artery
k. Carotid sinus
l. Pyramidal lobe (thyroid gland)
m. Trachea
n. Lymph node
o. External jugular vein
p. Left subclavian artery
q. Left subclavian vein
r. Arch of aorta

Concepts Application

System or Structure	Hyperthyroidism	Hypothyroidism
Weight	Weight loss	Weight gain
Emotional state	Nervous; irritable	Lethargic; disinterested
Temperature preference	Prefers cool climate	Prefers warm climate
Hair	Fine hair with hair loss	Coarse hair that breaks easily
Skin	Warm skin with hyperpigmentation	Coarse, dry, scaling skin at pressure points
Neck	Goiter	No goiter
Gastrointestinal	Increased peristalsis; increased frequency of bowel movements	Decreased peristalsis; constipation
Eyes	Puffiness in periorbital region	Proptosis; lid retraction

Case Study

1. Data deviating from normal: Patient complains of severe recurring headache. Nasal stuffiness occurs with headache. Nothing seems to help headache.
2. Get more information about the headache, including the following:

   Pattern of headaches: How often do the headaches occur? At what time of day do they occur? How would you characterize the onset of the headaches (gradual vs. sudden)?

   Characteristics of headache: Where is the pain? What is the pain like? How long does the pain last? How severe is the pain?

   Precipitating factors: What brings the headache on?

   Treatment: What has Rob done to try to treat these headaches?

   History: Is there any past or recent history of trauma to the head?
3. Assess range of motion in the neck, if possible, and attempt to palpate the neck for lymph nodes.

Critical Thinking

1. Percussion of the head and neck is not routinely performed. Percussion over the sinuses is applicable if the examiner suspects sinusitis in order to determine whether tenderness exists. There is also some evidence that individuals with hyperparathyroidism have a low-pitched sound to percussion of the skull (as opposed to a high-pitched sound, which is normally expected).
2. Similar to percussion, auscultation of the head is not routinely performed. However, if a vascular anomaly of the brain is suspected, bruits might be heard. It is best to listen over the eyes, the temporal region, and just below the occiput of the skull.

Content Review Questions

Multiple Choice

1. c
2. b
3. d
4. d
5. a
6. b
7. d
8. a
9. d
10. b
11. d
12. a
13. c
14. d
15. a

CHAPTER 11

Application to Clinical Practice

Matching 1

1. c
2. b
3. e
4. a
5. d
6. f

Concepts Application 1

Structure	What Should Be Examined
1. Eyelid	Observe position of the eyelids when the eyes are open and when the eyelids are closed completely. Inspect for eversion or inversion of the eyelids and the presence of nodules.
2. Conjunctiva	Inspect for inflammation, presence of foreign body, and increased erythema or exudate. Observe for pterygium.
3. Cornea	Assess corneal sensitivity. Note lipid deposits on cornea. Assess clarity.
4. Iris and pupil	Check for response to light and accommodation. Estimate pupillary sizes; compare them for equality.
5. Lens	Inspect for clarity—lens should appear transparent.
6. Sclera	Check for color of sclera and for pigmentation.
7. Lacrimal apparatus	Inspect and palpate. Check for tearing.

Concepts Application 2

1. a. Location: Lesion is 2 DD at clock position of 2:00
   b. Length: 2/3 DD
   c. Width: 1/3 DD

Matching 2

1. f, c
2. g, d
3. a
4. b
5. h, e

Case Study

1. Data deviating from normal: History of poorly controlled diabetes; sudden change in vision; significant visual acuity findings; ophthalmoscope findings; new vessels and presence of hemorrhage vessels
2. Ask the patient whether he has pain. Ask whether the change in vision has been gradual and progressive or intermittent. Ask whether he has any other symptoms associated with the change in vision, such as intolerance to light. Ask him whether he currently wears contact lenses or glasses. Ask how long he has had diabetes.
3. It is important to determine the previous visual acuity results to compare with the current one.
4. Andy has one major problem at this point that affects multiple areas. If he loses his vision, the impact on functional abilities will be tremendous and will include (but not be limited to) safety, self-care activities, management of his diabetes, independence, and employment.

Critical Thinking

1. General inspection of external structures of the eye should be done. Visual acuity should be checked with a Snellen E chart. A red reflex should be checked; corneal light and reflex and cover–uncover should also be done. Finally, examination of extraocular movements and cranial nerves III, IV, and VI should be done, including asking the child to follow through the six cardinal fields of gaze.

2. The first clue is the size; retinal arteries are about one fourth narrower than retinal veins. The second difference is the color. Arteries appear as a very light red color and may have a narrow band of light reflex in the center. Veins, on the other hand, are darker in color and do not have a band of light reflex.

Content Review Questions

Multiple Choice

1. d
2. b
3. c
4. b
5. a
6. c
7. d
8. a
9. c
10. b
11. c
12. a
13. a
14. d
15. b
16. b
17. b
18. c
19. b
20. a

CHAPTER 12

Application to Clinical Practice

Matching

1. c
2. b
3. d
4. a
5. g

6. i
7. h
8. f
9. e

Anatomy Review

a. Auricle
b. External auditory canal
c. Tympanic membrane
d. Stapes and footplate
e. Eustachian tube
f. Round window
g. Oval window
h. Cochlea
i. Cochlear and vestibular branch
j. Facial nerve
k. Semicircular canals
l. Incus
m. Malleus

Clinical Application

1. Koplik spots
2. Darwin tubercle
3. Malocclusion
4. Epstein pearls

Case Study

1. Data deviating from normal: Fever; complaints of ear pain; presence of drainage in ear canal; tympanic membrane perforation; reduction of hearing in left ear; quiet affect; limited talking
2. Ask what treatment the child has received for the ear pain from the medicine man in the past. Ask the mother whether she has ever seen drainage from the ear with past problems. Ask whether the child has been treated at a hospital or clinic for ear pain in the past.
3. If possible, complete a Rinne test. A full hearing assessment with an audiometer is probably in order as well. Also, complete a developmental assessment.
4. Primary problems: The child has obvious hearing impairment. There is also some evidence of a possible developmental delay, perhaps associated with the hearing loss.

Critical Thinking

1. To differentiate redness associated with crying versus otitis media, look for other clinical signs, primarily bulging and mobility of the tympanic membrane.

Content Review Questions

Multiple Choice

1. a
2. c
3. b
4. a
5. d
6. c
7. a
8. c
9. a
10. b
11. d
12. b
13. b
14. c
15. d

CHAPTER 13

Application to Clinical Practice

Auscultation Sounds

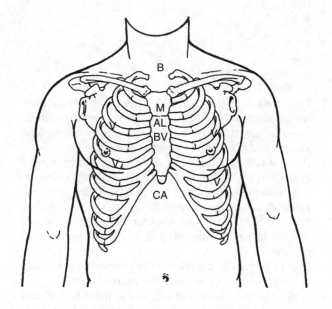

Examination Technique

Finding	Examination Method	Finding	Examination Method
Biot respiration	Inspection	Bronchial	Auscultation
Tactile fremitus	Palpation	Rhonchi	Auscultation
Cheyne-Stokes respiration	Inspection	Barrel chest	Inspection
Dullness	Percussion	Hyperresonance	Percussion
Vesicular	Auscultation	Wheezes	Auscultation
Tympany	Percussion	Tracheal tug	Palpation
Dyspnea	Inspection	Crackles	Auscultation
Bronchophony	Auscultation	Diaphragmatic excursion	Percussion
Vibration	Palpation	Bronchovesicular	Auscultation
Kussmaul breathing	Inspection	Crepitus	Palpation

Matching

1. d
2. j
3. h
4. g
5. b
6. i
7. f
8. c
9. e
10. a

Case Study

1. Data deviating from normal: History of shortness of breath; limitation in activity; interrupted sleep (requiring pillows); smoking history; labored breathing with tachypnea; presence of cyanosis; underweight with protruding ribs; increased anteroposterior diameter; reduced chest wall movement; diminished tactile fremitus; adventitious breath sounds; diminished breath sounds
2. Ask about chest pain with shortness of breath. Ask about the presence of cough. Ask how old the patient was when she started smoking and how long she has been smoking as much as she currently is.
3. Assess oxygen saturation, body weight, and rhythm of breathing pattern. Assess for presence of retractions. Percuss the chest for tone and diaphragmatic excursion.
4. Primary problems for this patient include respiratory or oxygenation problems and nutrition problems. Patients who are short of breath have difficulty maintaining adequate nutrition.

Critical Thinking

1. He has a 9-year history at one third pack a day (3 pack years), a 15-year history at half pack a day (7½ pack-years), and a 32-year history of 1 pack a day (32 pack-years) for a total of a 42½ pack-year history.

2. These symptoms are consistent with tuberculosis. High-risk groups include Native Americans or American Indians and immigrants from Mexico. He should be placed in airborne isolation until a diagnosis is made.
3. Ask what has changed. The mother said the family moved recently; ask about the new home and environment, as well as possible irritants within the new home. Also ask about ventilation, air conditioning, and exposure to smoke and pets in or around the home.

Content Review Questions

Multiple Choice

1. d
2. c
3. b
4. d
5. a
6. c
7. a
8. a
9. c
10. d
11. c
12. a
13. b
14. a
15. c
16. b
17. d
18. b
19. d
20. b
21. b
22. c
23. a
24. d
25. b

181

CHAPTER 14

Application to Clinical Practice

Anatomy Review

a. Brachiocephalic artery
b. Superior vena cava
c. Coronary sulcus
d. Right coronary artery
e. Right atrium
f. Anterior cardiac veins
g. Right ventricle
h. Apex
i. Left ventricle
j. Left coronary artery
k. Great cardiac vein
l. Left atrium
m. Left pulmonary artery
n. Arch of aorta
o. Left subclavian artery
p. Left common carotid artery

Concepts Application

Valve	Where Would You Auscultate?
Tricuspid valve	Fourth left intercostal space
Mitral valve	Fifth left intercostal space
Aortic valve	Second right intercostal space
Pulmonic valve	Second left intercostal space

Matching

1. g
2. i
3. c
4. d
5. e
6. j
7. a
8. h
9. b
10. f

Case Study

1. Data deviating from normal: Shortness of breath; fatigue that interferes with routine activities; sleeping difficulty; labored breathing with elevated respiratory rate, pulse rate, and blood pressure; pitting edema in lower extremities; frothy-looking phlegm
2. Complete a symptom analysis on the shortness of breath and fatigue. Ask the patient whether he has symptoms associated with chest pain, cough, or nocturia. Ask the patient about cardiovascular history.
3. Perform a precordial assessment, including inspection, percussion, palpation, and auscultation.
4. First, this patient has a perfusion problem. The decrease in cardiac output reduces the perfusion of oxygenated blood to the body, causing the symptoms of fatigue. Second, this patient has an oxygenation problem. Because the heart is not pumping efficiently, blood is backing up in the pulmonary bed, resulting in pulmonary edema. Pulmonary edema interferes with the exchange of oxygen and carbon dioxide in the lungs.

Critical Thinking

1. This finding, without other symptoms, may not be relevant. However, children who have congenital heart defects tend to squat frequently because squatting relieves dyspnea.
2. Look for polyarthritis, chorea, erythema marginatum, subcutaneous nodules, arthralgia, an increase in the sedimentation rate, and leukocytosis.
3. Diabetes causes an increase in basement membrane of capillaries, which makes these vessels narrower. Narrowing contributes to hypertension and impaired perfusion of the lower extremities.

Content Review Questions

Multiple Choice

1. c
2. b
3. a
4. a
5. c
6. a
7. c
8. c
9. c
10. b
11. b
12. c
13. c
14. a
15. a
16. c

17. a
18. b
19. d
20. c
21. a

22. d
23. d
24. b
25. c

CHAPTER 15

Application to Clinical Practice

Anatomy Review

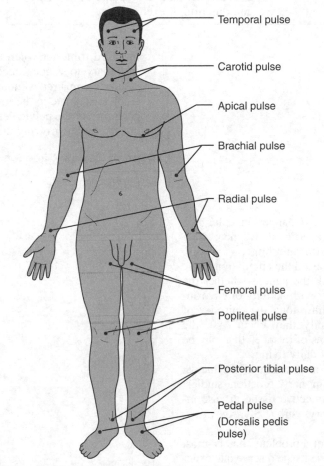

From Sorrentino SA, Remmert LN: *Mosby's Essentials for Nursing Assistants,* ed 5, Mosby, St. Louis, 2014.

Concepts Application 1

Location of Pain	Probable Obstructed Artery
Calf muscles	Superficial femoral artery
Thigh	Common femoral artery or external iliac artery
Buttock	Common iliac artery or distal aorta

Concepts Application 2

Arterial Insufficiency	Venous Insufficiency or Musculoskeletal Disorders
1. Pain comes on during exercise.	Pain comes on during or often several hours after exercise.
2. Pain is quickly relieved by rest.	Pain is relieved by rest but sometimes only after several hours or even days. Pain tends to be constant.
3. Intensity increases with intensity and duration of exercise.	Intensity of pain has greater variability than arterial pain in response to intensity and duration of exercise.

Matching

1. d
2. e
3. b
4. c
5. h
6. g
7. a
8. f

Case Study

1. Data deviating from normal: Changes in color and temperature of the hands; exertional dyspnea; presence of dark lesion on the fifth right finger
2. Complete a symptom analysis on the circulation in the hands and the dyspnea. Ask the patient whether the pain and color changes vary with activity or environmental changes; also ask how long the episodes of pain last and how frequently they occur. Ask the patient about other symptoms of dyspnea that may be interfering with activities of daily living.
3. Perform further neurologic assessment of the hands; obtain chest film and pulmonary function studies; complete evaluation for connective tissue disease including appropriate laboratory work (ESR, ANA titer, and chemistry studies).
4. This patient has a circulatory problem that is most likely secondary to connective tissue disease and exacerbated by smoking. The intermittent spasms of the arterioles in the fingers cause pallor, and the accompanying decrease in circulation produces claudication. The appearance of impending ulceration on the finger signals the need for monitoring of the patient's circulatory status. The patient may develop spasms in the nose and tongue, and she should be educated about this possibility and encouraged to report any changes in her circulatory status.

Critical Thinking

1. The symptoms suggest venous thrombosis, and the patient is at risk for pulmonary embolus.
2. Blood pressure can change with position changes by the mother. Hypotension is frequently noted during the third trimester when the patient is supine. This is secondary to venous occlusion of the vena cava and resulting impaired venous return. In addition, blood tends to stagnate in the lower extremities as a result of occlusion of the pelvic veins and the inferior vena cava created by the growing uterus.

Content Review Questions

Multiple Choice

1. c
2. b
3. a
4. c
5. b
6. c
7. b
8. c
9. c
10. a
11. a
12. c
13. a
14. b
15. d
16. c
17. a
18. d
19. b
20. c

CHAPTER 16

Application to Clinical Practice

Matching

1. d
2. e
3. b
4. a
5. c
6. h
7. g
8. f

Concepts Application

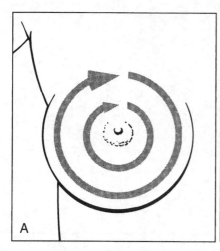

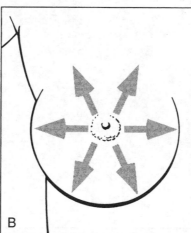

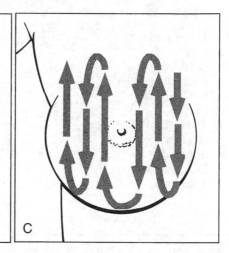

Case Study

1. Data deviating from normal: Patient has a history of a nontender breast lump, noticeable for about 9 months. Mass has increased in size over 9 months. Risk factors include early onset of menarche and the fact that the patient is childless. Palpable lump is present in the left upper outer quadrant. Dimpling noted on left breast. Left nipple is retracted. Bloody discharge is noted from nipple when squeezed.
2. Ask about personal or family history of breast disease. Ask the patient whether she does regular breast self-examinations. Ask whether she has ever had a mammogram. Ask about location of the lump. Ask whether the lump is tender now. Ask whether she has noticed nipple discharge. Ask about changes in the lump size in relation to her menstrual cycle.
3. Inspect the areolae. Besides location, the following characteristics must be assessed with a breast mass: size, shape, consistency, tenderness, mobility, and borders. Palpate the axilla. It is especially important to note any lumps or masses in the left axilla.
4. Primary problems: This patient has a very suspicious breast mass consistent with malignancy. She also seems to be in denial about this problem.

Critical Thinking

1. Risk factors for breast cancer: Patient is female. She is older than 40 years of age. She had an early onset of menarche. She had her first and only child at the age of 36 years. She has a strong family history of breast cancer. Although it cannot be predicted who will and will not develop breast cancer, this woman certainly has very strong risk factors.
2. Offer the following instructions: Perform breast self-examination at the same time every month. Undress and stand in front of a mirror. Look at your breasts in the following three positions: (1) standing with hands on hips, (2) standing with arms extended above your head, and (3) leaning forward with your hands outstretched. Watch for any changes in the way your breast appears, such as a dimpling, puckering, or changes in size. Palpate your breasts. Raise your left arm over your head. Starting at the nipple of the left breast, firmly press the fingers from your right hand in a circular motion, working outward and feeling every part of your breast. Feel for any lump or mass. After you palpate your breast, squeeze the nipple and look for any discharge. Repeat this procedure with the other breast. You may do this procedure standing or lying down. If you feel any lumps or see any discharge from your nipple, contact your primary health provider.

Content Review Questions

Multiple Choice

1. a
2. c
3. a
4. b
5. a
6. c
7. c
8. b
9. d
10. b
11. d
12. b
13. a
14. b
15. d
16. a
17. b
18. a

Application to Clinical Practice

Anatomy Review

a. Liver
b. Gallbladder
c. Ascending colon
d. Small intestine
e. Cecum
f. Appendix
g. Bladder
h. Sigmoid colon
i. Descending colon
j. Transverse colon
k. Stomach
l. Spleen

Matching 1

1. d
2. c
3. a
4. e
5. f
6. b

Concepts Application 1

Structure	Quadrant	Region
Appendix	Right lower quadrant	Right inguinal
Colon	Ascending or transverse right upper quadrant	Ascending—right lumbar
	Transverse and descending left upper quadrant	Transverse—umbilical
	Ascending right lower quadrant, descending left lower quadrant	Descending—left lumbar
Gallbladder	Right upper quadrant	Right hypochondriac
Liver	Right upper quadrant	Right hypochondriac (right lobe) Epigastric
Pancreas	Left upper quadrant (body)	Epigastric
	Right upper quadrant (head)	Left hypochondriac (tail)
Small intestine	Right lower quadrant	Umbilical
	Left lower quadrant	Hypogastric
Spleen	Left upper quadrant	Left hypochondriac
Stomach	Left upper quadrant	Epigastric Umbilical

Concepts Application 2

Condition	Type of Pain	Abdominal Signs	Associated Symptoms or Findings
Peritonitis	Sudden or gradual onset of generalized or localized pain described as dull or severe; increased pain with deep inspiration	+ Markle sign + Rosving sign + Blumberg sign	Shallow respirations; nausea and vomiting; guarding; decreased bowel sounds; + obturator and iliopsoas tests
Cholecystitis	RUQ and epigastric pain that refers to right subscapular region	+ Murphy sign	Anorexia, nausea, vomiting, fever, abdominal rigidity
Ectopic pregnancy	Lower quadrant pain that may refer to the shoulder; agonizing pain with rupture	+ Cullen sign + Kehr sign	Tender cervix, discharge, dyspareunia, symptoms of pregnancy, spotting, hypogastric tenderness, mass on bimanual pelvic examination; with rupture: shock, rigid abdominal wall distention
Pancreatitis	Sudden and dramatic LUQ, umbilical, or epigastric pain that may be referred to left shoulder	+ Grey-Turner sign + Cullen sign	Fever, epigastric tenderness, vomiting
Renal calculi	Intense flank pain extending to groin and genitals	+ Kehr sign	Fever, hematuria

Concepts Application 3

Sounds of Auscultation	Possible Associated Condition
Increased bowel sounds	Gastroenteritis, early intestinal obstruction, or hunger
High-pitched tinkling sounds	Intestinal fluid and air under pressure early obstruction
Decreased bowel sounds	Peritonitis and paralytic ileus
Friction rub	Inflammation of the peritoneal surface from tumor, infection, or infarction
Venous hum	Increased collateral circulation between portal and systemic venous systems

Matching 2

1. e
2. h
3. c
4. i
5. g
6. d
7. a
8. j
9. f
10. b

Case Study

1. Data deviating from normal: Abdominal pain (progressively worse); loss of appetite and nausea; guarded position; hot skin, possibly indicating fever; absence of bowel sounds; pain to palpation and guarding RLQ; positive rebound tenderness in RLQ
2. Ask the patient about vomiting with her nausea. Ask about her menstrual cycle, about the possibility of pregnancy, and about bowel elimination and the appearance of her stool.
3. Check vital signs (of particular interest is temperature). Auscultate for arterial bruits and venous hums. Percuss kidney for costovertebral angle tenderness. Perform iliopsoas muscle test and obturator muscle test.
4. Primary problems: Patient demonstrates symptoms consistent with acute abdominal condition, very likely appendicitis. A complete blood count would be helpful.

Critical Thinking

1. Listen to the abdomen for bruits in the aortic, renal, iliac, and femoral arteries. A bruit in these arteries may indicate stenosis or an aneurysm. Listen in the umbilical area for a venous hum (soft, low pitched, and continuous). A venous hum suggests increased collateral circulation between portal and systemic venous systems and may indicate portal hypertension. A friction rub is high pitched and may be heard in association with respiration. This may indicate inflammation of peritoneal surface from tumor or infection.
2. Ask Mr. Cane to place his hand on top of his abdomen. You will then place one of your hands on the side of his abdomen near the flank; use the other hand to tap on the other side of the abdomen. The test result is considered positive if the tap causes a fluid wave through the abdomen that is felt by your hand on the side of his abdomen.

3. Expected findings unique to pregnancy include decreased bowel sounds, linea nigra, striae, diastasis recti, quickening, and venous pattern.

Content Review Questions

Multiple Choice

1. d
2. c
3. b
4. c
5. a
6. d
7. b
8. c
9. c
10. d
11. d
12. d
13. d
14. b
15. a
16. a
17. c
18. c
19. a
20. b
21. c
22. a
23. b
24. c
25. d

CHAPTER 18

Application to Clinical Practice

Anatomy Review

a. Prepuce of clitoris
b. Frenulum of clitoris
c. Labium minus
d. Lesser vestibule of Skene duct opening
e. Greater vestibule of Bartholin duct opening
f. Vestibule
g. Fourchette
h. Posterior commissure
i. Perineum
j. Anus

187

k. Fossa navicularis
l. Hymen
m. Vaginal orifice
n. Labium majus
o. Vestibule
p. Urethral or urinary orifice
q. Glans of clitoris
r. Anterior commissure
s. Mons pubis

7. C
8. O, E
9. E
10. C

Matching 1

1. O, E
2. C
3. O, E
4. E
5. C
6. O, C

Matching 2

1. d
2. e
3. a
4. f
5. g
6. b
7. c

Concepts Application

Position	Description	Advantages or Disadvantages
Knee–chest	Patient lies on side with both knees bent with top leg closer to chest.	May be difficult or uncomfortable for patient who is obese or has very large breasts.
Diamond shape	Patient lies on back with knees bent so legs are spread flat and heels meet at the foot of table.	Patient must be able to lie flat on back for this position and have flexible legs.
Obstetric stirrups	Patient lies on back near foot of bed with legs supported under the knees in obstetric stirrups.	These offer more support than the traditional foot stirrups.
M-shape	Patient lies on back, knees bent apart, feet resting on the examination table close to buttocks.	Entire body can be supported by the table.
V-shape	Patient lies on back with legs straightened out and spread wide to either side of the table.	Assistance is needed to maintain this position.

Case Study

1. Data deviating from normal: History suggests some type of acute inflammation. History is also suggestive of multiple sex contacts; primary partner has multiple sex contacts. Mass with inflammation, discharge, and extreme pain to palpation needs further evaluation.
2. Ask patient about sexual history and associated medical problems, if any. Identification of protection (or lack of) would also be helpful.
3. A culture of discharge should be obtained for evaluation. If patient is too uncomfortable for internal examination, this may need to be delayed until the inflammation has resolved.
4. Based on symptoms and findings, the patient most likely has an acute abscess of the Bartholin gland. This is frequently associated with gonococcal or staphylococcal infection.

Critical Thinking

1. The key concept when performing an examination on a patient with a visual impairment is to explain everything that is to occur, as well as what you want the patient to do. Before the examination, the patient should be given an opportunity to explore the instruments used during the examination. Other general concepts to keep in mind include introducing yourself, remembering to identify others who enter the room, and letting the patient know when others are leaving the room. Also, orient the patient to the surroundings. This patient may need assistance in getting into the proper position for examination.
2. The history is vital to obtain. At this age, it is necessary to talk with her while her parents are out of the room. Questions should be simple, gentle, and nonjudgmental. These will greatly improve the accuracy of the information she is willing to share. There is no

one set rule to determine the age when a full examination of the genitalia is necessary. However, a good rule of thumb is that if the patient is sexually active, then an examination should be done. The examination should be carried out similarly to that of an adult.

Content Review Questions

Multiple Choice

1. c
2. a
3. b
4. b
5. a
6. d
7. b
8. c
9. d
10. b
11. b
12. a
13. d
14. d
15. b
16. b
17. d
18. c
19. a
20. c

CHAPTER 19

Application to Clinical Practice

Anatomy Review

a. Rectum
b. Seminal vesicle
c. Levator ani muscle
d. Ejaculatory duct
e. Anus
f. Bulbocavernosus muscle
g. Glans
h. Testis
i. Urethra
j. Corpus spongiosum
k. Corpus cavernosum
l. Prostate gland
m. Symphysis pubis
n. Urinary bladder

Matching 1

1. d
2. b
3. e
4. a
5. c

Matching 2

1. c
2. d

3. a
4. b
5. e

Case Study

1. Data deviating from normal: Protrusion or mass is noted in left groin area. History suggests a possible hernia.
2. Discuss the patient's level of discomfort and other related symptoms. Determine whether there is history of this problem.
3. Examiner needs to determine whether this hernia is reducible. If it is nonreducible, it may require prompt surgical intervention. Also, full examination of the genitalia is in order.
4. Based on symptoms and findings, the patient most likely has a direct inguinal hernia.

Critical Thinking

1. Discuss why genital self-examination is done: to screen for testicular cancer and to identify sexually transmitted infections. Discuss how to perform genital self-examination. This should include the following: inspection of the tip for evidence of swelling, sores, or discharge; palpation of the entire shaft of the penis from the base to the glans to feel for lumps or tenderness; and examination of the scrotum for color, texture, and presence of lesions. The patient should also palpate his scrotum for the presence of lumps, swelling, or tenderness.
2. Be sure one of the child's parents is present. Explain to the child what you must do and why (to be sure all his body parts are healthy). It may be necessary for the parent to reassure the child that it is OK for the examiner to see his "privates."

Content Review Questions

Multiple Choice

1. d
2. a
3. c
4. b
5. b
6. c
7. a
8. c
9. a
10. a
11. c
12. c
13. d
14. b
15. d
16. b
17. c
18. d
19. a
20. c

Application to Clinical Practice

Anatomy Review 1

a. Superior rectal valve
b. Internal hemorrhoidal plexus
c. Internal sphincter
d. Superficial external sphincter
e. Anal crypt
f. Subcutaneous external sphincter
g. Perianal gland
h. Rectal sinus
i. Rectal column
j. Deep external sphincter
k. Levator ani muscle
l. Inferior rectal valve
m. Middle rectal valve

Anatomy Review 2

a. Prostate gland
b. Utricle
c. Opening of Cowper gland
d. Cowper gland
e. Ejaculatory orifice

Matching

1. b
2. f
3. d
4. g
5. a
6. e
7. c

Concepts Application

Screening Method	What It Reflects	What Results Mean	When It Is Indicated
DRE	The size and character of the prostate gland	Cancer with prostate may feel hard and have irregular nodules.	Part of periodic health screening for all men older than 50 years old and in men older than 40 years old with positive risk factors.
PSA	Glycoprotein produced by prostate tissue	PSA <4 ng/mL: normal PSA <4 to 10 ng/mL: borderline PSA >10 ng/mL: high The higher the PSA level, the more likely cancer exists. However, men with prostate CA can have borderline to low results.	PSA routine screening in conjunction with DRE in all men older than 50 years old and in men older than 40 years old with positive risk factors.
PSA velocity	Measurement of rising PSA level over time	Rapid rise of PSA levels may suggest prostate cancer.	Used when PSA level is in the borderline range.
Free PSA ratio	Measurement of the ratio of unbound (free) to bound PSA	A low unbound (free) PSA ratio suggests an increased chance that prostate cancer is present.	Used when PSA level is in the borderline range.
Biopsy	Sample of prostate tissue is taken for pathologic analysis	Normal tissue: no disease or benign enlargement. Abnormal or malignant tissue in presence of prostate CA.	Recommended when: (1) PSA level is in the high range, (2) PSA is in the borderline range with abnormal DRE findings, or (3) PSA is borderline with a low free PSA ratio.
TRUS	Ultrasonography of the prostate; can measure prostate volume and shape and size	Indicates areas of the prostate that require biopsy.	Used when PSA level is in the borderline range.

Case Study

1. Data deviating from normal: Sensation of rectal fullness; rectal bleeding; blood in stool; palpable mass in the rectum; weight loss; enlargement of prostate
2. Ask the patient about changes in bowel elimination pattern or changes in the appearance of the stools (besides presence of blood). Ask about abdominal discomfort or distention. Ask about problems with urination (problems with starting or force of stream). Ask about sexual history.
3. Examination should include guaiac test and inguinal lymph node assessment. As part of the abdominal assessment, the examiner should specifically consider the possibility of pelvic or abdominal masses.
4. The patient has an enlarged prostate and a rectal mass. They may be interrelated or completely independent of one another. Further diagnostic testing is indicated.

Critical Thinking

1. The symptoms have some similarity, but findings will be different.
   Acute prostatitis: The patient will have an inflamed prostate; therefore, the prostate will be tender, and the patient will likely have a fever. Symptoms of obstruction develop more quickly than with the other two problems. With palpation, the prostate will be tender and possibly asymmetric. Additionally, the seminal vesicles may be dilated and tender to palpation.
   Benign prostate hypertrophy: Symptoms will develop gradually, with complaints of hesitancy, decreased force of stream, dribbling, and incomplete emptying of the bladder. With palpation, the prostate will feel rubbery, symmetric, and enlarged.
   Prostatic carcinoma: The symptoms of obstruction gradually occur. With palpation, the prostate is hard and irregular and feels asymmetric; the median sulcus is obliterated.
2. Some of the questions you could ask include:
   When did bleeding start?
   How much bleeding have you noticed?
   When and where do you see the bleeding?
   What does the blood look like?

Do you have any other symptoms associated with the bleeding such as pain, gas, cramping, or weight loss? What do you think is causing the bleeding?

Content Review Questions

Multiple Choice

1. a
2. b
3. c
4. d
5. a
6. a
7. b
8. d
9. a
10. d
11. b
12. c
13. d
14. d
15. c
16. d
17. b
18. c
19. a
20. b

CHAPTER 21

Application to Clinical Practice

Matching 1

1. e
2. b
3. h
4. b
5. f
6. d
7. a
8. e
9. c
10. g

Concepts Application 1

Symptoms and Assessment Findings	Problems to Consider
Heberden nodes and Bouchard nodes noted on hands	Osteoarthritis
Low back pain that radiates to the buttocks and posterior thigh, with tenderness over the spine	Lumbar disk herniation
Heat, redness, swelling, and tenderness to the metatarsophalangeal joint	Gouty arthritis of the great toe
Subcutaneous nodules on the forearm near the elbow	Rheumatoid arthritis
Tenderness, swelling, and a boggy sensation with palpation along the grooves of the olecranon process; increased pain with pronation and supination	Epicondylitis or tendonitis
A child with muscle atrophy and symptoms of progressive muscle weakness	Muscular dystrophy
A child complaining of pain in the elbow and wrist; will not move his or her arm; maintains arm in a flexed and pronated position	Radial head subluxation

Matching 2

1. f
2. b
3. g
4. h
5. c
6. d
7. a
8. e

Case Study

1. Data deviating from normal: Diagnosis of RA; significant joint pain; limitations in self-care activities; limitations in socialization; difficulty with posture and gait; deformities to joints; tender, inflamed joints with palpation; subcutaneous nodules at the ulnar surface of the elbows
2. Ask the patient what medications she is taking for the RA. Find out whether she is involved with any other nonpharmaceutical therapies. Ask her whether these things help or make a difference. Ask whether she has any assistive devices that she uses or whether she receives any assistance with self-care activities.
3. The examiner should perform documentation of ROM in various joints. Use of a goniometer would be particularly helpful.
4. Self-care activities, pain, social isolation

Critical Thinking

1. Muscle strain results if a muscle is stretched or torn beyond its functional capacity. A sprain is a stretching or tearing of a supporting ligament of a joint. A fracture is a partial or complete break in the continuity of the bone. Because the injury involves the joint, muscle strain is not likely. Both fractures and sprains are associated with pain and swelling and can have a bluish discoloration, so it is not always easy to differentiate these. If Mark walked in bearing weight on the affected ankle, it is doubtful that a fracture resulted; if he was unable to bear weight at all, it could be a fracture or a severe sprain; thus, radiography is usually the final diagnostic indicator.
2. A dislocation of the radial head, or radial head subluxation, is caused by jerking the arm upward while the elbow is flexed. This can occur by someone pulling on a child's arms during play or even while dressing a child. The parents must understand how this injury occurred and be taught to avoid arm-pulling activities.

Content Review Questions

Multiple Choice

1. a
2. b
3. c
4. d
5. c
6. d
7. d
8. a
9. d
10. b
11. c
12. c
13. a
14. c
15. a
16. b
17. d
18. c
19. b
20. a

CHAPTER 22

Application to Clinical Practice

Anatomy Review 1

a. Pituitary gland
b. Optic chiasma
c. Hypothalamus
d. Corpus callosum
e. Cerebrum
f. Skin
g. Superior sagittal sinus
h. Thalamus
i. Skull
j. Dura mater
k. Galea aponeurotica
l. Tentorium cerebelli
m. Midbrain
n. Cerebellum
o. Pons
p. Medulla oblongata

Anatomy Review 2

a. Cerebrum
b. Thalamus
c. Hypothalamus
d. Cerebral peduncle
e. Cerebellum
f. Hypoglossal (XII)
g. Spinal accessory (XI)
h. Vagus (X)
i. Glossopharyngeal (IX)
j. Acoustic (VIII)
k. Facial (VII)
l. Abducens (VI)
m. Trigeminal (V)
n. Trochlear (IV)
o. Oculomotor (III)
p. Pituitary gland
q. Optic (II)
r. Olfactory (I)

Concepts Application 1

Examination Procedure	Cranial Nerve(s) Tested
Whisper test	CN VIII
Patient sticks out tongue and moves it from side to side	CN XII
Taste test with sugar, salt, and lemon	CN VII (anterior), CN IX (posterior)
Visual acuity	CN II
Patient puffs out cheeks and shows teeth	CN VII
Patient shrugs shoulders against examiner's hands	CN XI
Smell test with coffee, orange, and cloves	CN I
Eyes constrict and dilate in response to light	CN III
Patient clenches teeth (temporal muscles contracted)	CN V

Concepts Application 2

Age of Infant	Observed Response	Name of Reflex	Expected or Unexpected?
2 months	The infant demonstrates a strong grasp of the examiner's finger when it is placed in the infant's palm.	Palmar grasp	Expected; this should disappear by 3 months
4 months	When held in an upright position with the soles of the feet touching the surface of a table, the infant flexes the legs upward in a curled position and holds them there.	Stepping	Unexpected; although the age is appropriate, the expected observed response is an alternating flexion and extension of the legs.
6 months	With the child lying supine, turn the head to one side; the arm and leg extend on the side the head was turned toward.	Asymmetric tonic neck	Unexpected at 6 months
8 months	The infant abducts and extends the arms and legs in response to sudden movement of the head and trunk backward. The arms then adduct in an embracing motion, followed by relaxation.	Moro	Unexpected; this should disappear by 6 months of age

Matching

1. c
2. b
3. g
4. e
5. a
6. h
7. d
8. f
9. i

Case Study

1. Data deviating from normal: Patient has been diagnosed with CVA. He had a headache preceding the incident. Patient's history includes inability to talk. He has left-sided paresis. He requires assistance for mobility. Patient avoids eye contact and cries.

2. Ask Mr. Thomas whether he thinks he can swallow normally. Ask him whether he has any pain or discomfort. Ask Mrs. Thomas about her husband's medical and family history. Ask about medications Mr. Thomas may be currently taking. Ask Mrs. Thomas whether her husband lost consciousness or had a seizure with this incident.

3. Assess gag reflex. Test reflexes (deep tendon). Assess for drooling.

4. Patient has weakness on one side of his body, which affects nearly all aspects of functional abilities. He has problems with communication, nutrition, and mobility as well.

Critical Thinking

1. Kevin's findings are invalid because he did not adjust his tool to determine two-point discrimination. Different body surfaces have varying sensitivity; depending on what body surface is being tested, the distance between two points on the tool must be adjusted. For instance, on the fingertips, the minimal distance for the two points is 2.8 mm. On the chest and forearms, the minimal distance is 40 mm. Most body surfaces are not able to detect one point versus two points at 1 inch (2.5 mm) apart.

2. The frontal lobe is the primary motor cortex; thus, an infarction in this area will affect motor function primarily on the opposite side of the lesion. Because the patient has a left infarction, he will be affected on the right side. Additionally, if the Broca area is affected, the motor dysfunction will affect this patient's ability to form words.

Content Review Questions

Multiple Choice

1. c
2. a
3. b
4. d
5. c
6. c
7. b
8. b
9. a
10. b
11. c
12. c
13. d
14. d
15. d
16. a
17. c
18. a
19. d
20. a

CHAPTER 23

Application to Clinical Practice

Concepts Application

Examination Component	Recommended Elements of Examination
Medical history	Illnesses or injuries since the last checkup or PPE Hospitalizations or surgeries Medications used by the athlete (including those he or she may be taking to enhance performance) Use of any special equipment or protective devices during sports participation Allergies, particularly those associated with anaphylaxis or respiratory compromise and those provoked by exercise Immunization status, including hepatitis B and varicella *Height and weight**
Cardiac	Symptoms of syncope, dizziness, shortness of breath, fatigue, or chest pain during exercise History of high blood pressure, heart murmurs, arrhythmias Family history of heart disease (e.g., cardiomyopathies, long QT syndrome, Marfan syndrome, arrhythmias) Previous history of disqualification or limited participation in sports because of a cardiac problem *Blood pressure (sitting position, appropriate size cuff, repeated readings)* *Heart rate and rhythm* *Pulses* *Auscultation for murmurs*
Respiratory	Asthma, coughing, wheezing, or dyspnea with exercise
Neurologic	History of a significant brain injury or concussion Numbness or tingling in the extremities Severe headaches
Vision	Visual problems Corrective lenses *Visual acuity*

Examination Component	Recommended Elements of Examination
Orthopedic	Previous injuries that have limited sports participation Injuries that have been associated with pain, swelling, or the need for medical intervention *Screening orthopedic examination*
Psychosocial	Weight control and body image Dietary habits; calcium intake Stresses at home or in school Use or abuse of drugs and alcohol *Attention to signs of eating disorders, including oral ulcerations, decreased tooth enamel, calcium intake, edema*
Genitourinary	Age at menarche, last menstrual period, regularity of menstrual periods, number of periods in the past year, and longest interval between periods (athletic girls tend to experience menarche at a later age than nonathletic girls) *Palpation of the abdomen* *Palpation of the testicles* *Examination of inguinal canals*

Italics indicate physical examination items.

Critical Thinking

1. a. Stage 1 Hypertension
   b. Two additional blood pressure measurements should be obtained in the subsequent weeks. If his blood pressure is consistently elevated, an evaluation should be conducted for an etiology and for end-organ damage.
   c. Contact
   d. Medical history, cardiac, respiratory, neurologic, complex, vision, orthopedic, psychosocial, genitourinary
2. a. Complex
   b. Neuropsychological testing and consultation with a multidisciplinary team that includes a sports medicine physician with experience in concussion management

Content Review Questions

Multiple Choice

1. b
2. c
3. a
4. d
5. c
6. a
7. d
8. b
9. b
10. b
11. c
12. d
13. c
14. a
15. b

CHAPTER 24

Application to Clinical Practice

Matching

1. f
2. j
3. h
4. e
5. k
6. m
7. b, c
8. g
9. a
10. l
11. d, e
12. m
13. j
14. i
15. m
16. f
17. j
18. m

Concepts Application

Examination Area	Body Systems Examined
Upper extremities	Integumentary, cardiovascular, respiratory, lymphatic, musculoskeletal, neurologic
Anterior chest	Integumentary, cardiovascular, respiratory, lymphatic, musculoskeletal, breasts and axillae
Abdomen	Integumentary, gastrointestinal, cardiovascular, musculoskeletal, lymphatic, neurologic
Head and neck	Integumentary, lymphatic, neurologic, musculoskeletal, visual, auditory, nose and paranasal, mouth and oropharynx

Critical Thinking

1. The most significant modification necessary with this examination is communication. It is vital that the examiner explain what is to be done and how. Even though a visual acuity examination will not be necessary, inspection of the eyes is still applicable.
2. The examiner must maintain composure and express confidence. It is extremely important to identify this patient's concerns and needs through active listening and therapeutic discussion. It is important to be as precise as possible and to set limits as appropriate.

Content Review Questions

Multiple Choice

1. a
2. c
3. b

4. d
5. a
6. d
7. c
8. c
9. b
10. a
11. d
12. c
13. c
14. a
15. b

CHAPTER 25

Application to Clinical Practice

Concepts Application

Symptoms	Body Systems That Might Be Involved
Chest pain	Cardiovascular, pulmonary, musculoskeletal
Headaches	Neurologic, cardiovascular, visual, auditory
Abdominal pain	Cardiovascular, gastrointestinal, urinary
Pain in the legs	Musculoskeletal, neurologic, integumentary, cardiovascular

Matching

1. b
2. c
3. d
4. a

Critical Thinking

Matching

1. c
2. g
3. i
4. d
5. a
6. f
7. h
8. b
9. e

Concepts Application

Examination Data	Possible Problems
A 54-year-old woman with jaundice, abdominal pain, nausea, and weight loss. Has pain to abdominal palpation; positive bowel sounds. Liver slightly enlarged; admits to alcohol use.	Cholecystitis, hepatitis, pancreatitis, cirrhosis, hepatic malignancy
A 66-year-old man with a chief complaint of breathing difficulty. Has increased respiratory rate, low-grade fever, rales, productive cough; increased tactile fremitus bilaterally.	Pneumonia, pulmonary edema, empyema
A 13-week-old infant girl with fever, irritability, poor eating. Infant is dehydrated and has a temperature of 103.7°F; soft abdomen.	Otitis media, upper respiratory infection, gastroenteritis
A 19-year-old female college student with a chief complaint of pain when urinating. Describes frequency and urgency. Patient has temperature of 100.4°F; has constant pain in pelvic area; positive pain with fist percussion over left flank.	Urinary tract infection, pyelonephritis, sexually transmitted infection

Content Review Questions

Multiple Choice

1. b
2. d
3. d
4. a
5. b
6. d
7. c
8. a
9. c
10. a

CHAPTER 26

Application to Clinical Practice

Concepts Application 1

1. Subjective
2. Chief concern
3. SOAP
4. Illustration
5. Objective
6. Incremental grading
7. POMR
8. Health history
9. Physical examination

Concepts Application 2

Problem #	Onset	Problem	Date Resolved
1.	June 1998	Low back pain	Ongoing
2.	1977	IDDM—poor control	Ongoing
3.	May 1997	Cholecystitis	Resolved
4.	1997	Family history of ASHD	Ongoing
5.	1997	Family history of CRF	Ongoing

Case Study

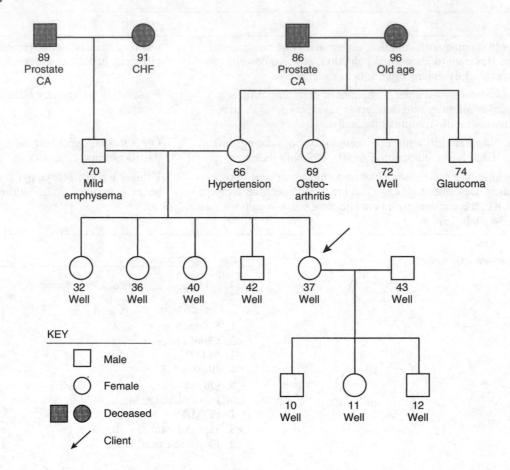

KEY

☐ Male

◯ Female

◼◕ Deceased

↙ Client

Critical Thinking

1. "OLDCARTS" refers to the following: O = onset of symptom; L = location of the symptom; D = duration of the symptom; C = character of the symptom; A = aggravating or associated factors of the symptom; R = relieving factors; T = temporal factors; and S = severity of the symptom.

2. Organs, masses, and lesions should be documented based on the following characteristics: texture or consistency; size; shape or configuration; mobility; tenderness; induration; heat; color; location; and other characteristics such as bleeding, discharge, and scarring.

Content Review Questions

Multiple Choice

1. a
2. d
3. c
4. b
5. d
6. a
7. c
8. d
9. c
10. a

Application to Clinical Practice

Concepts Application

1. Primary
2. Secondary
3. Secondary
4. Primary
5. Secondary
6. Secondary
7. Primary
8. Primary
9. Secondary
10. Secondary
11. Primary

Case Study

1. Findings:
   A: Has open airway; is moving air and is able to speak
   B: Respiratory distress; dyspnea with nasal flaring
   C: Circulation—has some cyanosis around lips; should palpate pulses
2. Administration of oxygen
3. Vital signs
4. Data deviating from normal: The respiratory data, dyspnea with bloody sputum, and blood gas findings. His neurologic and mental status suggests hypoxia. Significant fact is that he had knee surgery 2 weeks ago.
5. The most serious concern to continue to monitor for (and treat) is the respiratory status. A priority would be to manage the airway and provide ventilatory assistance because the laboratory findings indicate he does not have adequate ventilation. Chest radiography would be helpful.
6. This young man is in serious trouble, and if the respiratory status does not improve, death may follow. Initial data suggest an acute pulmonary embolus. Another problem to rule out is drug overdose.

Matching

1. b, e
2. d
3. a, f
4. c
5. f
6. b

Critical Thinking

1. a. Burns and being in a house fire should immediately alert any health care provider to the possibility of smoke, heat, and chemical inhalation. Injuries to the respiratory system may be the most significant injury these patients sustain.
   b. Young children and infants have small nasal and oral airway passages; shorter, narrower tracheas; and shorter necks. The larynx is higher and more anterior as well. These differences affect airway management. Children also have a large body surface area. Children who have sustained burns to the skin are more susceptible to fluid losses, hypothermia, and infection than are adults.

Content Review Questions

Multiple Choice

1. a
2. c
3. b
4. c
5. a
6. d
7. d
8. a
9. c
10. c
11. b
12. d
13. d
14. b
15. c